CW01368063

**IT'S OKAY
NOT TO
GET ALONG
WITH EVERYONE**

Also by Dancing Snail:
I'm Not Lazy, I'm on Energy Saving Mode

IT'S OKAY
NOT TO
GET ALONG
WITH EVERYONE

Dancing Snail

Translated by Sandy Joosun Lee

bl!nk

First published in the UK in 2025 by Blink Publishing
An imprint of Bonnier Books UK
5th Floor, HYLO, 105 Bunhill Row,
London, EC1Y 8LZ

Copyright © by Dancing Snail 2020
Published by arrangement with BACDOCI COMPANY., LIMITED
through Eric Yang Agency, Seoul, Korea

Translation copyright © Sandy Joosun Lee 2025

No part of this publication may be reproduced, stored or transmitted in any form or by any means, electronic, mechanical, photocopying or otherwise, without the prior written permission of the publisher.

The right of Dancing Snail to be identified as Author of this work has been asserted by her in accordance with the Copyright, Designs and Patents Act, 1988.

A CIP catalogue record for this book is available from the British Library.

Hardback ISBN: 978-1-78512-830-1

Also available as an ebook

1 3 5 7 9 10 8 6 4 2

Design and Typeset by Envy Design Ltd
Printed and bound in Lithuania

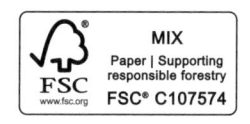

MIX
Paper | Supporting responsible forestry
FSC® C107574

Every reasonable effort has been made to trace copyright holders of material reproduced in this book, but if any have been inadvertently overlooked the publishers would be glad to hear from them.

The authorised representative in the EEA is
Bonnier Books UK (Ireland) Limited.
Registered office address: Floor 3, Block 3, Miesian Plaza,
Dublin 2, D02 Y754, Ireland
compliance@bonnierbooks.ie

www.bonnierbooks.co.uk

CONTENTS

PROLOGUE   9

PART 01 Not Too Close, Not Too Far

01 Intrusion into My Universe   14
02 'Oh Well' and 'Take It or Leave It'   18
03 Relationship Minimalist   22
04 It's Okay to Say You're Tired   25
05 How to Stop Acting 'Too Cool' and Start
    Being Considerate   28
06 Let's Stay Just This Close   30
07 Would You Mind Adjusting to Me?   33
08 The Freedom to Be Neither an 'Insider'
    Nor an 'Outsider'   39
09 You're Like a Hairpin – Never Around When
    I Need You   43
10 The Small Reasons Why Love Ends   46
11 The Right to Forget   48
12 To Someone I'll Never See Again   51
13 The 'Relationships Are Hard' Club   55
14 Emotional Hunger   58
15 Running into an Old Friend at a Wedding   60
16 The Opportunity Cost of Excitement   63

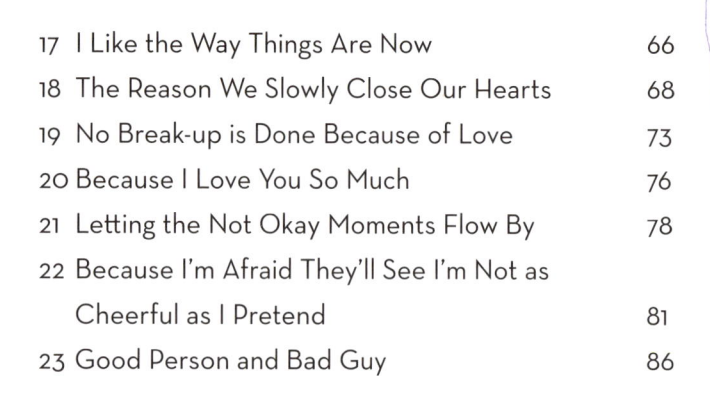

17 I Like the Way Things Are Now	66
18 The Reason We Slowly Close Our Hearts	68
19 No Break-up is Done Because of Love	73
20 Because I Love You So Much	76
21 Letting the Not Okay Moments Flow By	78
22 Because I'm Afraid They'll See I'm Not as Cheerful as I Pretend	81
23 Good Person and Bad Guy	86

PART 02 It's Okay Not To Get Along With Everyone

24 May You Never Be the Lesser in This World	92
25 Uncomfortable Means Uncomfortable	96
26 To Console Free from Comparison, to Celebrate Free from Anxiety	99
27 An Eye for an Eye, a Person for a Person	102
28 Between Stability and Passion	104
29 It's Okay to Be Uncool	108
30 To the Worrier Who Worries About Worrying	110
31 When It Doesn't Go Your Way, Go Your Heart's Way	113
32 Dry Comfort Over Forced Forgiveness	115
33 All the Emotions You Feel are Always Right	120
34 Same Moments, Different Memories	126
35 Trust the Relationship, Not the Person	128

36	Yes, I'm Lonely – But No, I Don't Want to Date	131
37	I Can Always Choose Better	137
38	I Stop Dwelling on Those Who Hurt Me	141
39	The Only One Who Can Embrace Me Unconditionally is Myself	144
40	I Don't Need to Be Liked by Everyone to Be Enough	149
41	Singlehood Compensation Bonus	154
42	Certain Things Can't Be Forced – The Human Heart Most of All	158
43	The Heart Locker	165
44	It's Okay Not to Be Whole on Your Own	169
45	If You Can Be Okay on Your Own	174

PART 03 People Always Need People

46	There's an Invisible Line Between You and Me	178
47	The Art of Being Not Too Close	182
48	The Right-sized Gap in the Heart	187
49	Somewhere Between Alone and Together	190
50	No One is Truly Indispensable	193
51	When Someone Enters Your Heart	197
52	When Excitement Alone Doesn't Feel Like Enough	199
53	When We're Meant to Cross Paths	202

54 Maybe, Just Once, It's Okay to Give My Whole Heart	204
55 Choosing to Let Go of the Time We Shared	207
56 Meaning of Friendship	211
57 People Always Need People	214
58 Taking a Step Back from Each Other's Lives	218
59 The Timeless Kind of Magic	223
60 Relationship is Not a Means for Happiness	226
61 How the Food Tasted, or the Breeze Smelled	230
62 We're So Alike!	232
63 There Are So Many Things More Important than Food	237
64 Letting Go of the Weight of Empty Connections	242
65 Simple Words But Full of Heart	247
66 Expanding Our Universe	250
67 Someone to Hold a Broken Piece of Your Heart	253

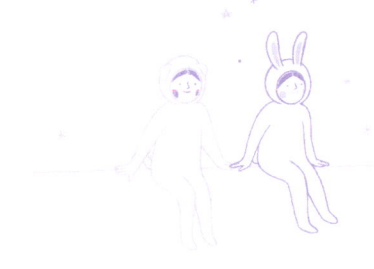

PROLOGUE

Ever since I was young I have always struggled to fit in. At school, I felt like a small drop of oil adrift in a sea of water, always floating and never blending in. I thought socialising would get easier as I grew older, but instead, it only got more complicated.

For instance, when should I stop replying to a text conversation? Is it appropriate to use emojis for work messages? Am I expected to attend the wedding of a friend I only keep in touch with once every year or two? How much condolence money is considered appropriate to give at a funeral? The questions only kept piling up in my head, like adding strokes of crayons onto fully painted canvas. When life gave me lemons, I wanted to go completely silent and not speak to anyone for a week. It was a clear sign that I had run out of social energy and needed a social detox.

Maybe I wasn't the only one who felt this way. Especially in this day and age, people seem to 'stan' cats and dogs (or even plants and inanimate objects) more than actual humans.

No matter how much I pretended to be fine on my own, I would inevitably confront the truth – that I am vulnerable and deeply dependent on others. It's a paradox, really. News of a celebrity's passing or a friend's wedding would still stir a subtle wave in my heart. We can never be completely unaffected by the lives of others, even those we have never met.

And even if people hurt us, we still crave the fulfilment that only human connection can provide. To protect myself from burnout and maintain balance, I've developed a few personal rules for navigating relationships. One of them I started following last year, which is 'I'm not obligated to see people I genuinely don't want to.' It sounds simple, but in practice, it comes with more considerations than one would expect. What defines an 'obligation' to meet someone? Where do you draw the line? If you start cutting people off, what if, in the end, no one is left around you? The more you struggle with that fear, the more critical it is to listen closely to your heart.

We live in an era of stress where the concept of 'small but certain happiness' – a phrase that refers to taking joy in life's simple, everyday pleasures – has been a thing for the past few years. But rather than accepting stress and figuring out a solution to release it, it turned out to be much more effective to avoid stressful environments in the first place. As part of that mindset, I've been trying out what I call 'minimalist relationships' –

cutting out people who negatively impact my mental health. I don't aim to be a good person to everyone. As long as I feel at peace with myself, I've decided not to worry too much about how others think of me. I've already spent too much of my life caring about how I looked through other people's eyes – time that chipped away at my self-esteem and even more time recovering from it. I've decided to break free from that cycle.

Now, I no longer try to be a 'good person' or to be loved by everyone. More than that, I want to focus my energy on living a happier life where I feel truly comfortable in my skin. I want to spend my time doing the work I love, meeting the people I love, writing about the things I love and creating art that I love. Life feels far more fulfilling to me when I minimise the time and energy spent on work I 'have to' do, people I 'have to' meet or writings and art I 'have to' complete.

    A friend of mine went on a diet where she drank two litres of water every day, only to get eczema on her hands. She saw a doctor, who explained that the sudden increase in water was likely the cause – her body couldn't properly process the excess water, so the water came out through her eczema. We jokingly laughed about it, wondering if that meant she had turned into a human humidifier. But later, it gave me a big life lesson: what works for others isn't necessarily what works for me.

    Depending on the people or situation, the type and

depth of relationships that feel like a 'comfortable place' can differ for everyone. It's okay to feel like an oil blot in a relationship that is meant to be like water. I don't need to change myself just to force a fit. I'd rather spend my energy meeting the people I want to see, not the ones I have to.

To my dearest family and friends – thank you for loving me from just the proper distance, and for embracing me just as I am, even when I'm not the warmest or most expressive. I'm deeply grateful.

Dancing Snail, June 2020

PART 01

NOT TOO CLOSE,
NOT TOO FAR

01
Intrusion into My Universe

No matter if the intentions were good,

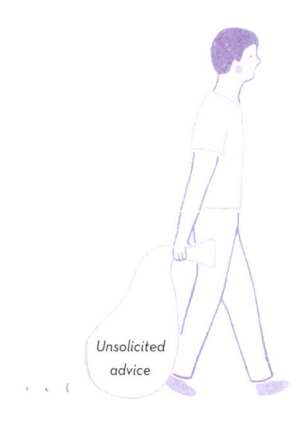

Unsolicited advice

when words cross the line into someone's privacy without their consent

I brought this because I care way too much to just let you keep doing ... whatever it is you're doing.

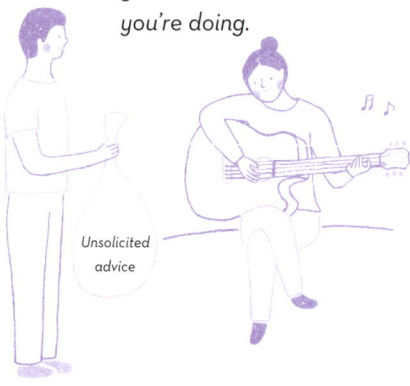

Unsolicited advice

they become nothing but unnecessary clutter.

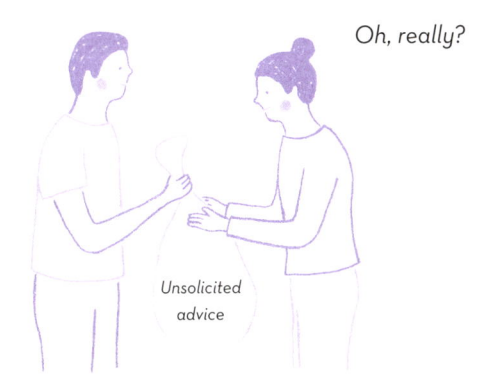

Oh, really?

Unsolicited advice

The best advice should always be given only when it's truly asked for.

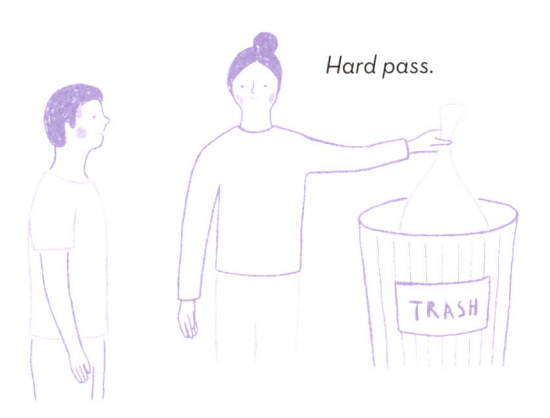

Hard pass.

TRASH

We need rooms of our own to focus on ourselves and preserve our identity and independence. There is a word for this in German: *spielraum*. But there is no direct equivalent in Korean. And when a concept doesn't exist in language, it often doesn't exist in reality either[1].

Perhaps this is why, in Korean culture, where the value of individual space tends to be underestimated, violations of that space seem especially frequent in daily life. On public transportation, it's common to see people 'manspreading' or pushing past strangers without consideration for others. In a society where such behaviours aren't necessarily seen as 'rude', it may explain why psychological boundaries are also less respected.

If a friend came over and, without asking, started rummaging through your fridge or flinging open the bedroom door, their visit would instantly cross the line into intrusion. Now imagine that same discomfort, not in your home but in your psychological world. Just as invading someone's physical space causes unease, forcing your thoughts onto someone else is a form of intrusion into their mental space. Even with the best of intentions.

---

1 Jung-woon Kim, *A Completely Different Time Flows in the Seaside Studio*, (21st Century Book, 2019)

Just as we should not intrude on others' physical space, we should watch our words and actions to avoid intruding on their emotional space. Timing is key in giving advice. Whether it is helpful or handy, if it is unsolicited, it's always better to hold it back.

02
'Oh Well' and 'Take It or Leave It'

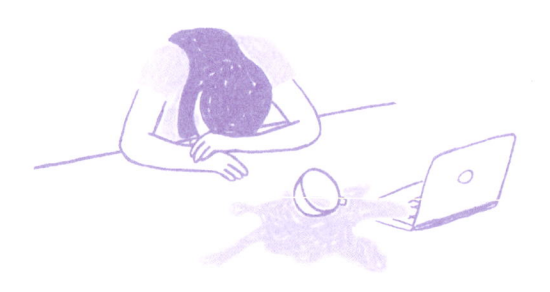

When nothing goes the way you wanted,

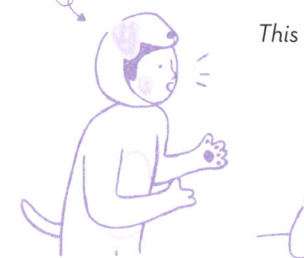

Weirdo

This weirdo shall also pass . . .

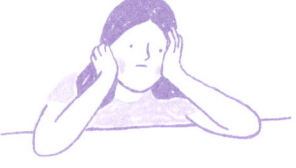

and even feeling disappointed in people just feels like a waste of energy

we need an 'Oh Well' mentality and a
'Take It or Leave It' attitude.

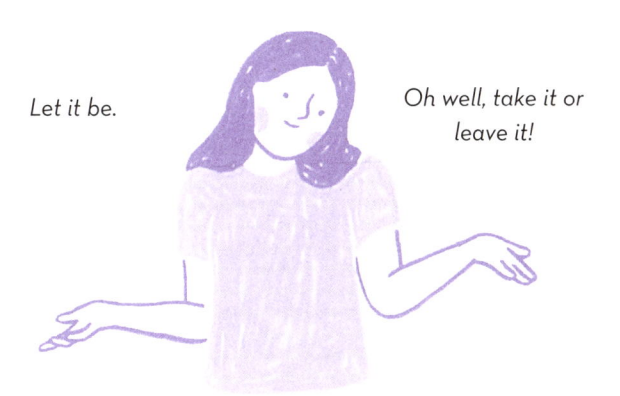

Let it be.

Oh well, take it or leave it!

We often find ourselves disappointed by those who don't turn out to be what we expected. This happens to everyone, but it's easy to lose faith in humanity when you're hit with wave after wave of disheartening news on social media or in the press. Sometimes, it can feel like you've developed an allergy to people altogether.

Maybe part of the blame lies with us because we set unrealistically idealistic expectations on those around us. Standards we ourselves can't even meet. When you get to know someone new, it's tempting to project your hopes onto them, to build them up into something other than they actually are. And while that optimism isn't inherently bad, it can make the eventual reality more discouraging. So, how do we keep going? How do we continue building and maintaining relationships while closing the gap between fantasy and reality?

One simple yet powerful mindset to adopt is what I call 'Oh Well' and 'Take It or Leave It'. These are ways to accept difficult situations or people with more humility, and also strategies to communicate your thoughts in a more level, respectful way. If you keep these two mindsets in your pocket, you can keep your peace of mind even when dealing with strange or unreasonable people – though of course, depending on how extreme they are, it might take a bit more time.

MY LITTLE TIPS FOR BALANCING HEALTHY BOUNDARIES IN RELATIONSHIPS

When someone lets you down, or things don't go as planned, say to yourself, 'Oh well.' And when you do need to speak up, end it with a tag: 'Take it or leave it.' Having these two phrases in your mental toolkit can help you navigate your relationships with less resentment and more peace. That way, you won't get sick of humanity.

03
Relationship Minimalist

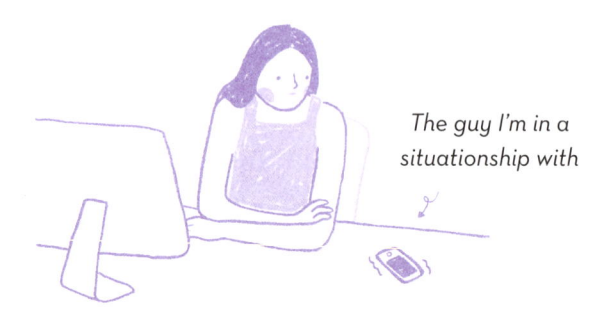

The guy I'm in a situationship with

When you're unsure about how you really feel about someone,

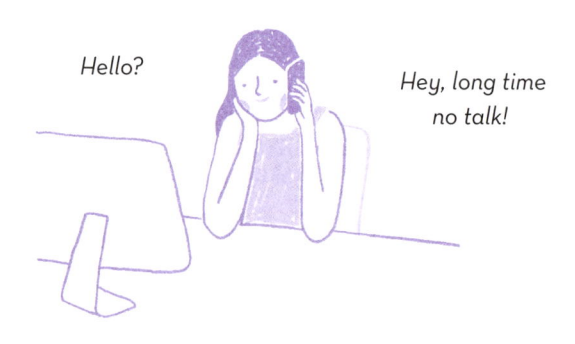

Hello?

Hey, long time no talk!

one of the clearest ways to find out is this:

Wait, this Saturday? Where?

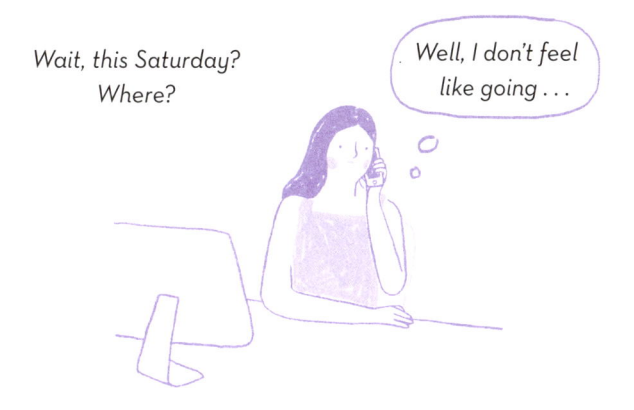

Well, I don't feel like going...

Does their smallest invitation feel worth getting up for?

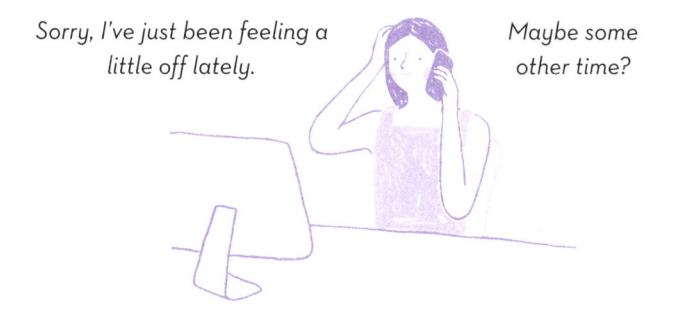

Sorry, I've just been feeling a little off lately.

Maybe some other time?

It's about keeping a 'laziness barometer' in your mind and paying attention to what it tells you.

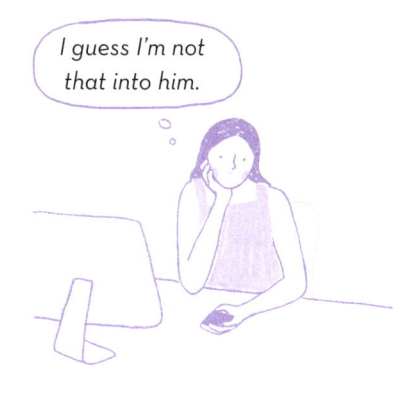

I guess I'm not that into him.

When it comes to re-evaluating relationships, I've found that laziness – or more precisely, a feeling of reluctance – is often the most telling litmus test. People are surprisingly willing to go out of their way for people they genuinely like, even if it involves effort or inconvenience. We gladly make plans, send messages and find excuses to meet. But what if you can't even muster the energy to decide whether it's worth spending time with someone? What if the thought itself feels like too much? That might be your mind's way of saying: it's time to let that person go.

We live in a world where focus and intention are more valuable than ever. 'If it doesn't spark joy, let it go' – the mantra popularised by tidying expert Marie Kondo – applies to people as much as possessions. Instead of clinging to half-hearted connections out of habit or guilt, maybe it's time to embrace the mindset of a relationship minimalist – someone who chooses depth over breadth, clarity over clutter.

So, here's a simple starting point: your phone. Are there unanswered messages quietly piling up in your inbox, each one a tiny weight of obligation? Begin with those. Sometimes, the people we delay responding to are the ones we've already emotionally moved on from.

04
It's Okay to Say You're Tired

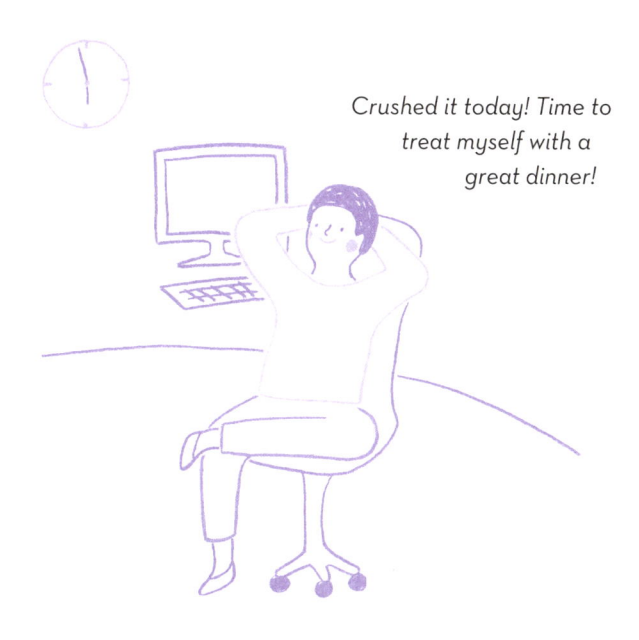

Crushed it today! Time to treat myself with a great dinner!

If today felt fulfilling and peaceful,

I still have some work to do. Goodnight!

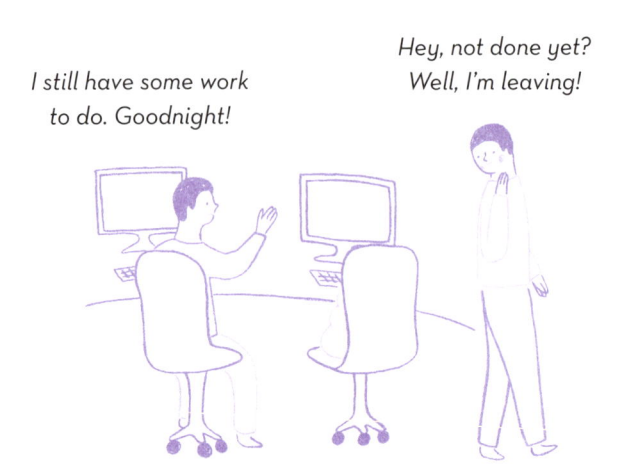

Hey, not done yet? Well, I'm leaving!

chances are, someone else made a big effort behind the scenes to make that possible.

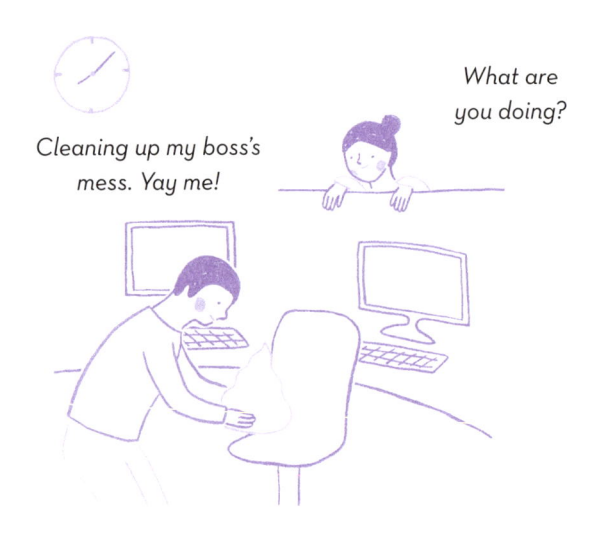

Cleaning up my boss's mess. Yay me!

What are you doing?

My peaceful day could never exist without someone's kindness and consideration.

There was a time when the phrase 'The Law of Conservation of Jerks' made the rounds online. The idea is simple: every group contains a fixed proportion of jerks, and when one disappears, someone else, who seemed perfectly normal before, suddenly steps in to fill the void. So, if you ever find yourself thinking, 'There are no jerks around me,' chances are, you might be the one.

As much as it makes us laugh, there's real psychological truth behind this joke. In any group dynamic, we tend to view the world through the lens of our comfort. People who are used to being on the receiving end of consideration often fail to notice when others are uncomfortable, simply because they assume, 'If I'm comfortable, everyone else must be too.' On the flip side, those who are naturally considerate tend to be more sensitive to others' discomfort, precisely because they themselves often feel it. Their empathy grows from experience.

This is why the most self-centred people – those we often label as 'jerks' – struggle to recognise when someone is extending kindness or suffering quietly. They're not necessarily trying to be inconsiderate; they're just not attuned to anything beyond their own experience.

So, if we find ourselves constantly adjusting for others – making space, keeping the peace, carrying the emotional load – it's okay to speak up. If we're going to extend kindness, we might as well make it clear we're doing it. Saying, 'This is hard for me' or 'I need a little help too' isn't selfish – it's actually a shortcut to getting mutual care and respect.

05
How to Stop Acting 'Too Cool' and Start Being Considerate

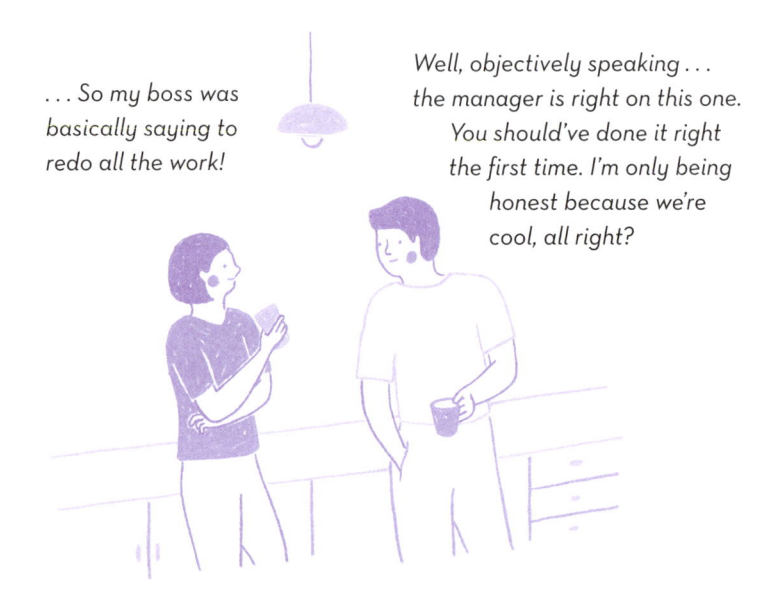

... So my boss was basically saying to redo all the work!

Well, objectively speaking... the manager is right on this one. You should've done it right the first time. I'm only being honest because we're cool, all right?

1. Recognise that being blunt under the guise of 'being cool' can actually hurt someone.

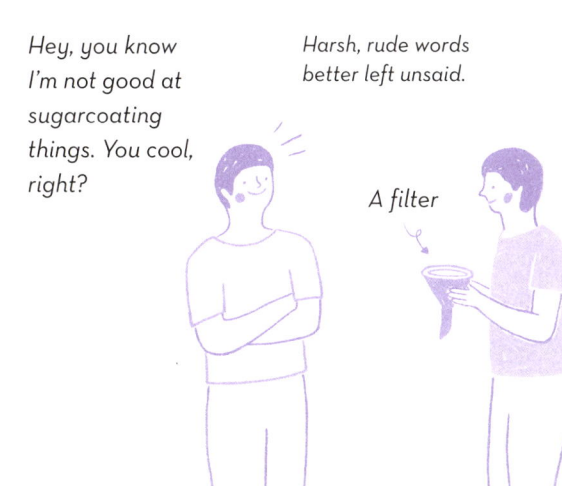

Hey, you know I'm not good at sugarcoating things. You cool, right?

Harsh, rude words better left unsaid.

A filter

So I thought . . . maybe your brain could use a little something—

2. If you say whatever you want without a filter, don't expect people to understand you.

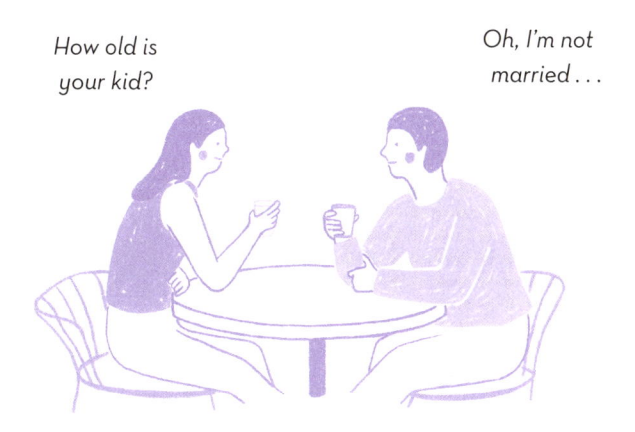

How old is your kid?

Oh, I'm not married . . .

3. Before you speak, ask yourself if your question might be crossing a line.

06
Let's Stay Just This Close

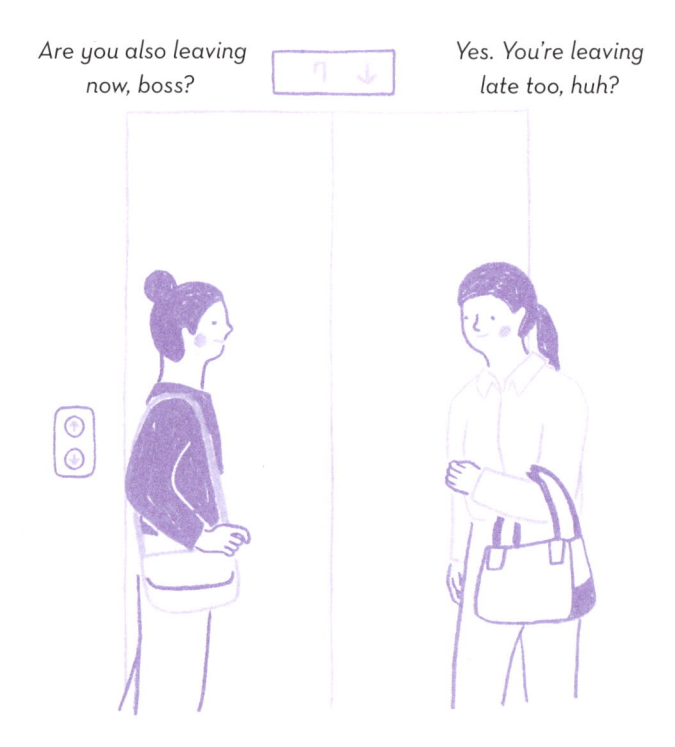

Are you also leaving now, boss?

Yes. You're leaving late too, huh?

I want to be liked.

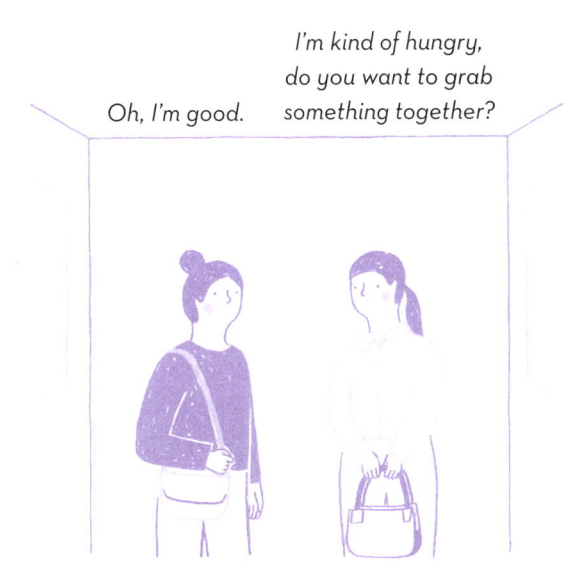

                    I'm kind of hungry,
                    do you want to grab
  Oh, I'm good.   something together?

I want to get closer.

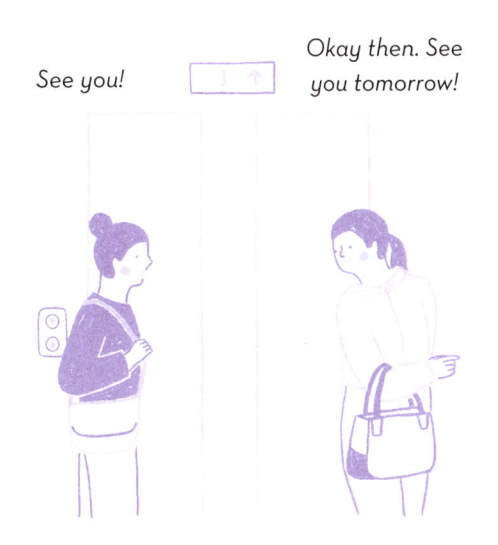

                        Okay then. See
  See you!   you tomorrow!

But not too close.

I've come to believe that no matter how close you get, work colleagues can never truly become personal friends. That's because the version of myself at work and the one when I'm around friends are entirely different. I consciously draw boundaries between the two, out of concern that revealing too much of my emotional side might unintentionally affect my career. (It's a lesson learned from overstepping those boundaries a few times already.)

As a freelance illustrator and writer, I often find myself in contact with people from publishing houses. One day, I learned that some authors are incredibly close with their editors. Seeing those warm, almost personal business connections made me wonder if I was keeping too much distance in my interactions with my editors. It's not that I necessarily want that kind of closeness, but strangely, I still felt a bit envious. That, in turn, made me question myself: Am I being too stiff? Too cold? The whole thing left me feeling conflicted. But no matter how much I think it over, I know that, given my personality, getting that close to someone I work with would still make me uncomfortable.

I do want to grow closer – but not too close. So let's stay at this comfortable distance.

07
Would You Mind Adjusting to Me?

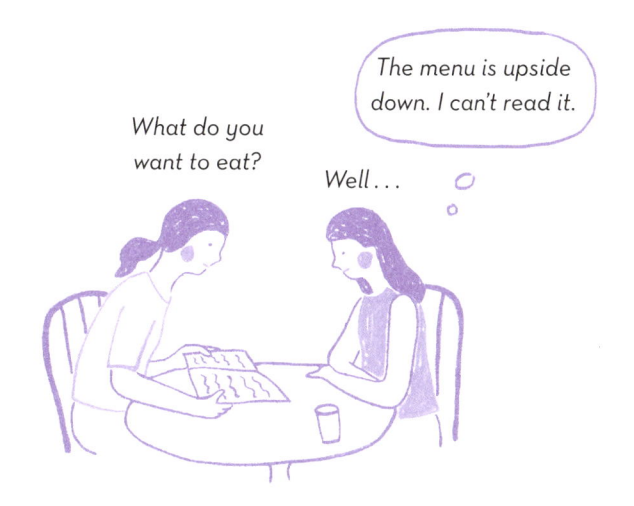

What do you want to eat?

Well . . .

The menu is upside down. I can't read it.

Some people not only expect others to adjust to them,

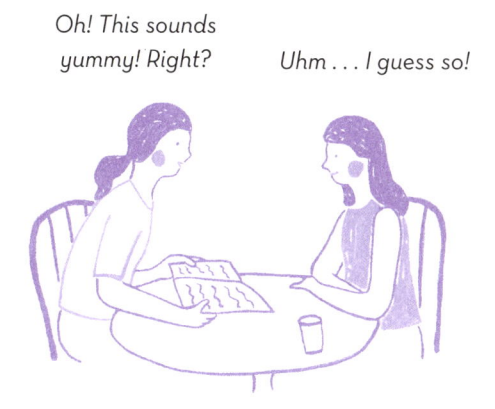

Oh! This sounds yummy! Right?

Uhm . . . I guess so!

but also take it for granted.

We'd like to have this!

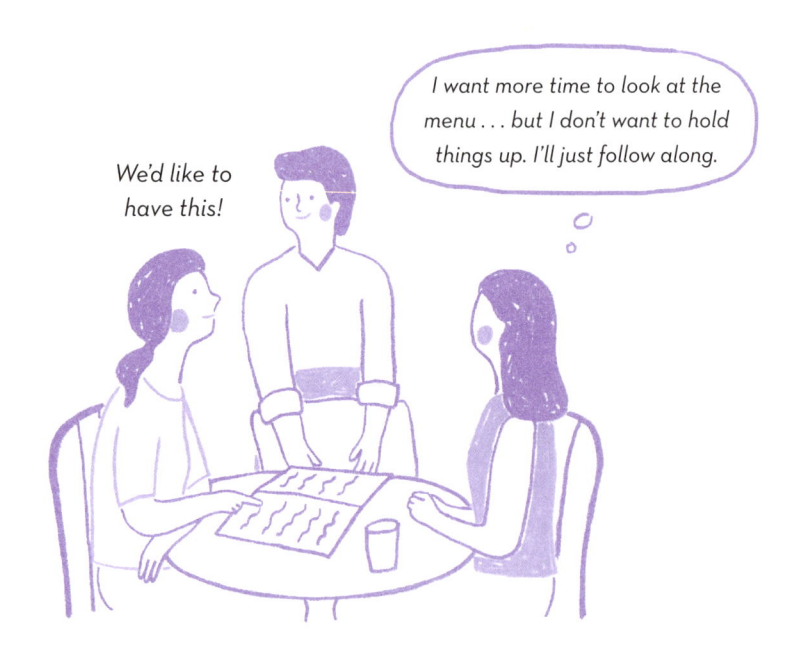

I want more time to look at the menu... but I don't want to hold things up. I'll just follow along.

And there are some people who actually feel more comfortable adjusting to others.

I'm so full! Should we go for a walk?

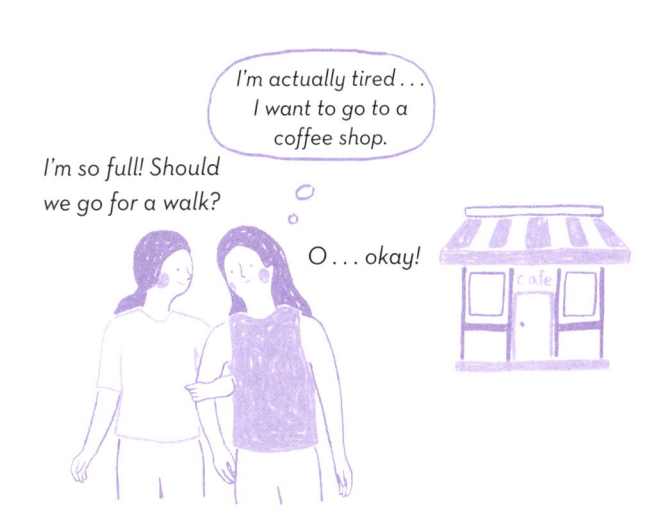

I'm actually tired... I want to go to a coffee shop.

O... okay!

When you constantly suppress your own needs to just go along with others,

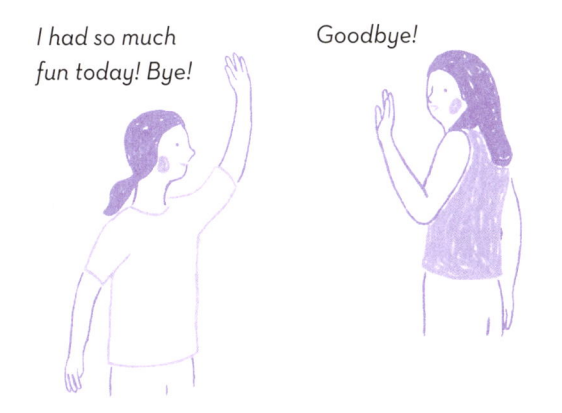

I had so much fun today! Bye!

Goodbye!

you're not giving them a chance to try adjusting to you in return,

Home sweet home.

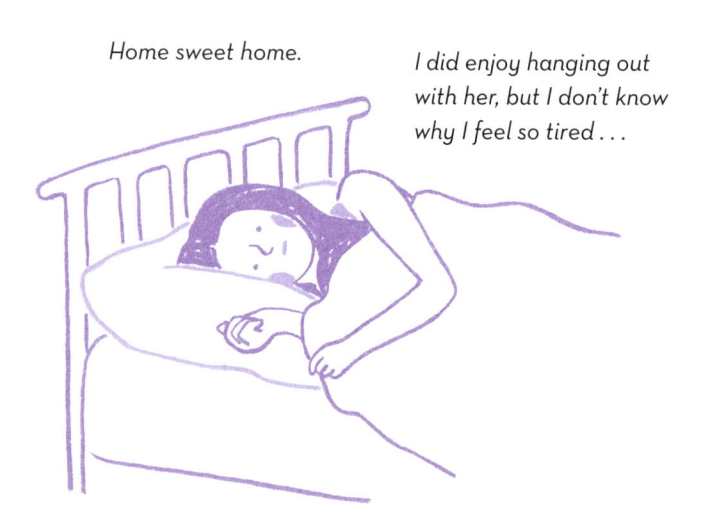

I did enjoy hanging out with her, but I don't know why I feel so tired . . .

let alone truly getting to know who you are yourself.

I once watched a video interview by a foreigner titled 'Struggles of Living in Korea' out of curiosity. But I was genuinely shocked when they said, 'At coffee shops, I ordered in Korean, but they responded in English. They don't even give you a chance to practise Korean.'

Looking back, I, too, would instinctively speak English when a foreigner asked me something. I was only nervous about whether my English was good enough to give them the right answer. It never crossed my mind to expect them to learn or speak Korean. To me, speaking English was an act of consideration. But I've come to realise that our definitions of what it means to be considerate might not be the same.

It wasn't just with foreigners. With most people – except for those I was extremely close to – I found it easier to accommodate their ideas and requests. As a first-born daughter, I think I was raised with the belief that the highest virtue was 'putting others first'. It became my most familiar, perhaps the only, mode of communication that I grew accustomed to. Over time, I began to conflate that habit with being considerate. As if yielding was a favour I was giving, when actually it was my default mode. A mental trap I created for myself.

As a result, it only increased my emotional fatigue and my desire for reciprocity, while the relationships didn't grow any deeper. After all, we had never once made a real effort to meet each other's needs.

What you think is 'being considerate' might not always be received the way you intended. So why not, once in a while, be honest about what you truly want? It gives the other person a real chance to be considerate of you. That kind of honesty might actually be what sustains a relationship in the long run. Because unless you speak up and show what you genuinely need, no one will ever know.

08
The Freedom to Be Neither an 'Insider' Nor an 'Outsider'

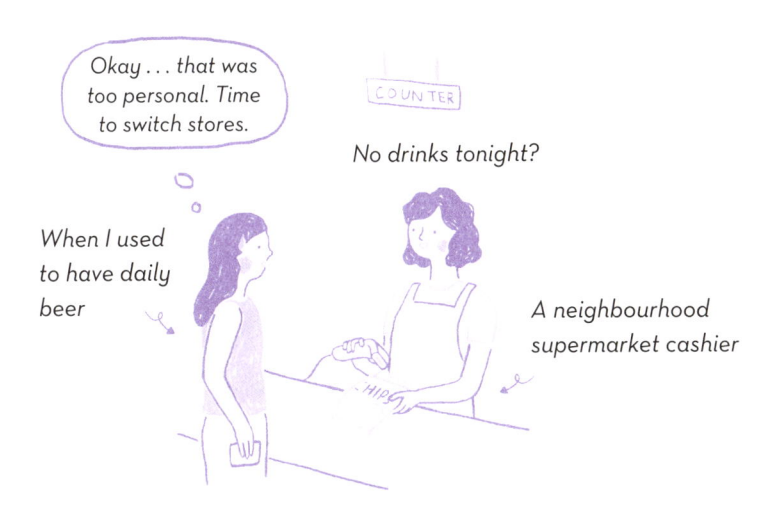

Okay ... that was too personal. Time to switch stores.

When I used to have daily beer

No drinks tonight?

COUNTER

A neighbourhood supermarket cashier

Too much attention feels overwhelming,

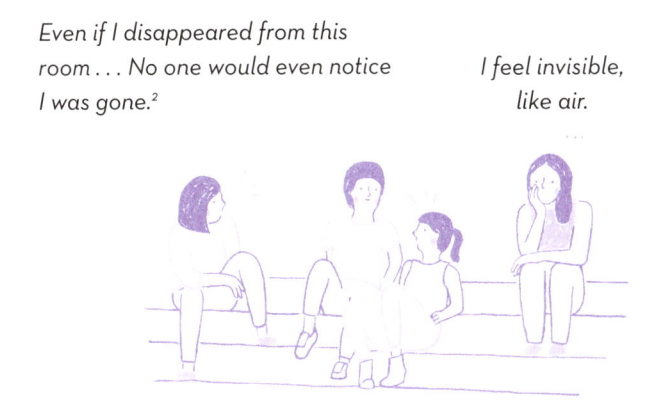

Even if I disappeared from this room ... No one would even notice I was gone.[2]

I feel invisible, like air.

but being invisible isn't what I want either.

---

2 Hyukoh, Panda Bear (single), released January 21, 2015

I love the glam but hate the gaze.

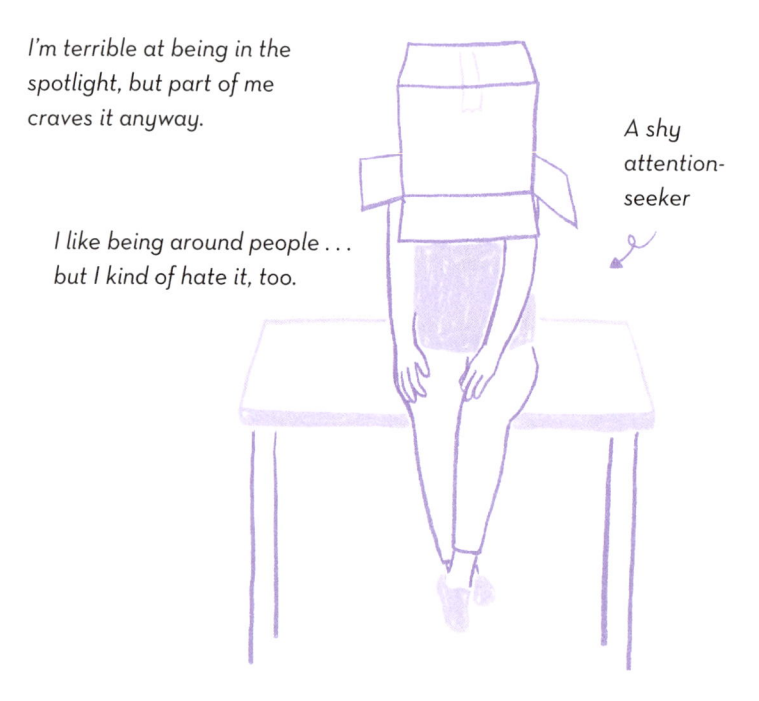

I'm terrible at being in the spotlight, but part of me craves it anyway.

A shy attention-seeker

I like being around people . . . but I kind of hate it, too.

So I live somewhere in between – not quite an insider, not quite an outsider.

I am a shy person – but one who still needs regular attention. You might call it a 'shy attention-seeker'. Sometimes, I find myself feeling a little jealous of *inssa* types (short for 'insiders'), but that doesn't mean I want to become one. I subtly seek attention from others, but the moment that attention actually lands on me, it becomes overwhelming – I just want to disappear. What's even more ironic is that when I encounter someone much more reserved than I am, I often feel compelled to take the first step and want to break that invisible boundary.

I don't think it's just me, but most people constantly shift parts of their personality depending on who they're interacting with or the situations they're in. It's because when more than two people engage, a 'flow of relationship' begins to emerge. (In psychology, this is referred to as 'group dynamics'.)

Consider the American movie *Her*, for instance – a love story between a human and AI. The relationship between Theo and the AI OS, Samantha, unfolds like a subtle game of tug of war. Their constant push and pull creates the rhythm – the flow – of their relationship. Through this process, Samantha begins to outgrow her initial programming, mimicking and learning from Theo's emotional intelligence. When even an AI OS can evolve through relational dynamics, it stands to reason that my own personality and behaviour are also fluid – shaped and reshaped within relationships.

The same is true for a 'flow of attention'. We navigate a delicate balance between being seen and being overlooked – between visibility and invisibility – throughout our lives. This process isn't always enjoyable, but it may be undeniable that it adds depth and colour to our experiences.

> **MY LITTLE TIPS FOR BALANCING HEALTHY BOUNDARIES IN RELATIONSHIPS**
>
> There's nothing strange about the feeling of wanting to move closer when someone pushes you away, and wanting to pull back when someone comes too close. Rather than trying to fit into a fixed role – whether as an *inssa* or *assa* (outsider) – or labelling yourself one way or another, maybe it's okay to just drift freely, finding your own rhythm in the sea of relationships around you.

09
You're Like a Hairpin – Never Around When I Need You

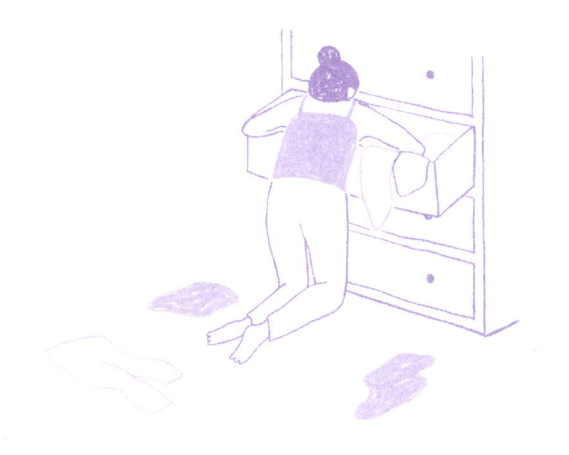

There are things that are always around when you don't need them, and gone the moment you do.

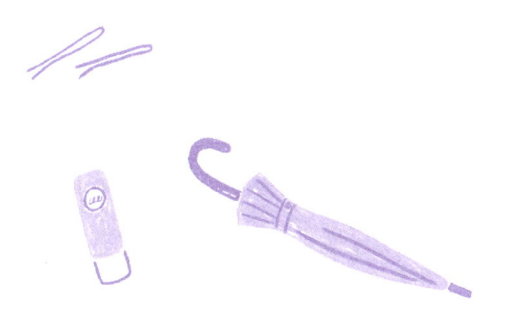

Hairpins, lip balm, umbrellas and . . .

You. The most unreachable when I need the most.

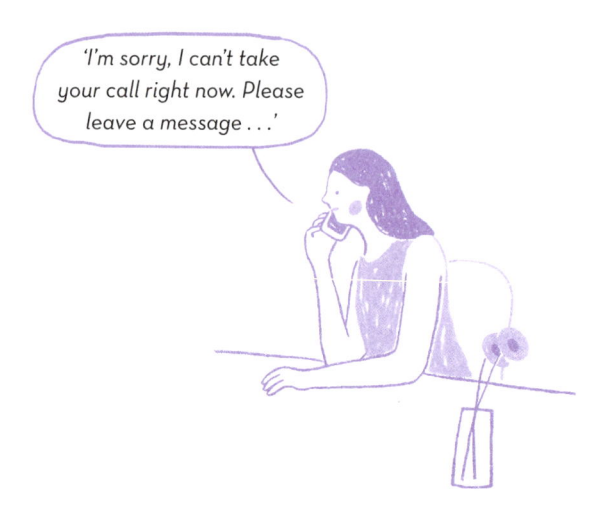

'I'm sorry, I can't take your call right now. Please leave a message...'

If you can't be there when I need you, how is that any different from not being there at all.

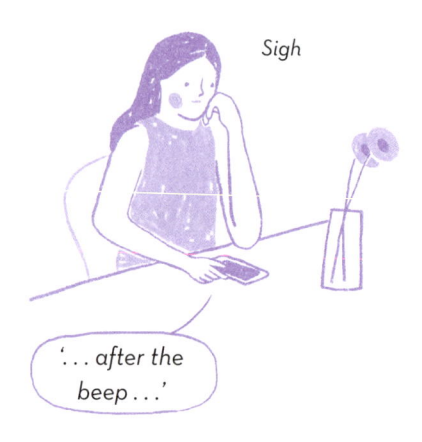

Sigh

'...after the beep...'

When a hairpin has been lying around for days, but suddenly goes missing the moment when you actually need it, you can't really say it's done its job. Same with relationships. Some people are like hairpins - always seemingly around, until the moment you need them. And then, they're nowhere to be found. When he needs me, I'm always easy to reach. But when I need him, somehow, he's never around. And if I ever bring up how that makes me feel, he treats me like I'm too emotionally dependent. Ugh. At least a hairpin doesn't make me feel lonely.

Just like it's hard to feel grateful for a hairpin that only rolls around when you don't need it, it's hard to appreciate someone who's never around when it counts. So don't feel like you have to work so hard to hold on to such people. Because someone who's never there when you need them might as well not be there at all.

10
The Small Reasons Why Love Ends

Love begins

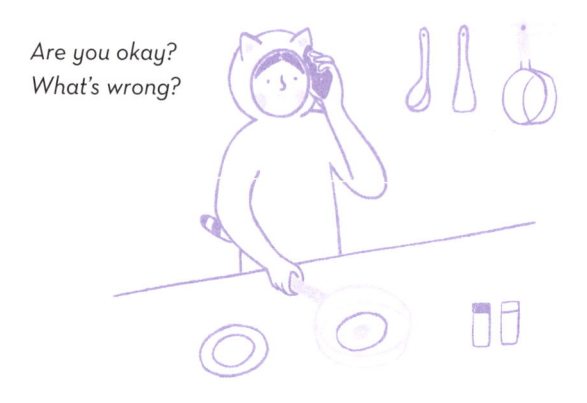

Are you okay? What's wrong?

with little things,

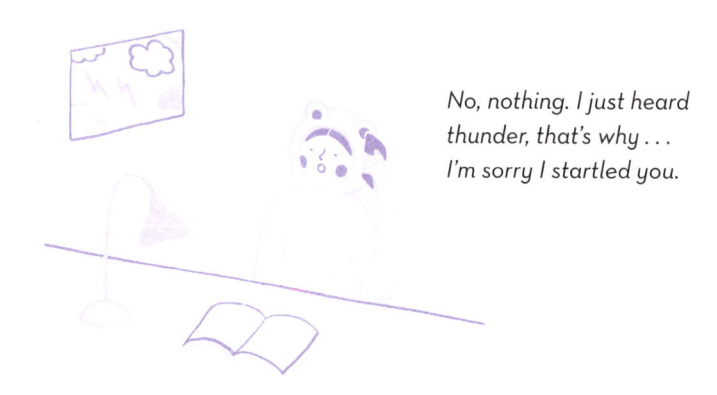

No, nothing. I just heard thunder, that's why . . . I'm sorry I startled you.

and ends

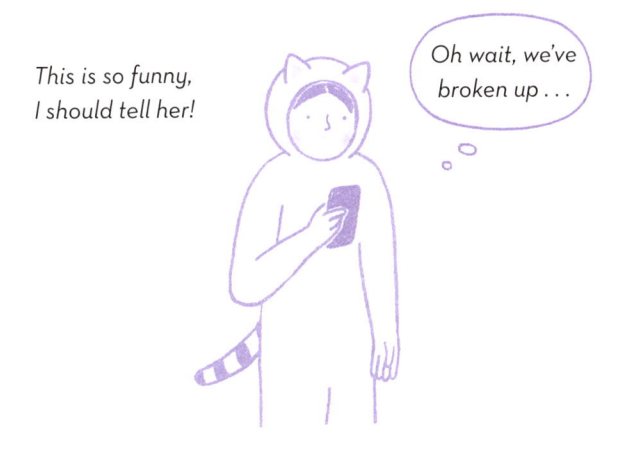

This is so funny, I should tell her!

Oh wait, we've broken up . . .

for small reasons.

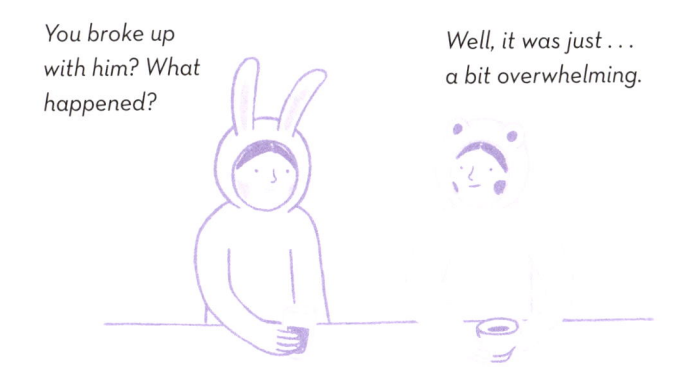

You broke up with him? What happened?

Well, it was just . . . a bit overwhelming.

11
The Right to Forget

I was doing just fine,

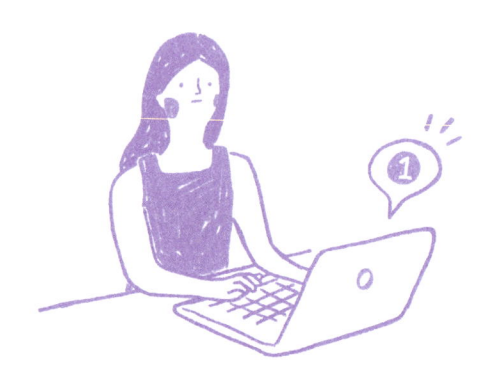

until a single notification turned my whole day upside down.

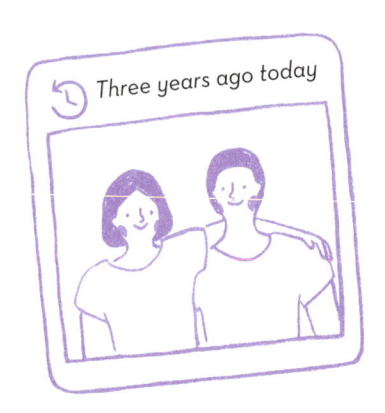

Three years ago today

What I hate even more than seeing you doing well

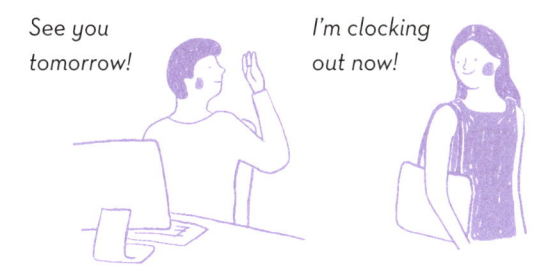

See you tomorrow!

I'm clocking out now!

is realising how much I still care.

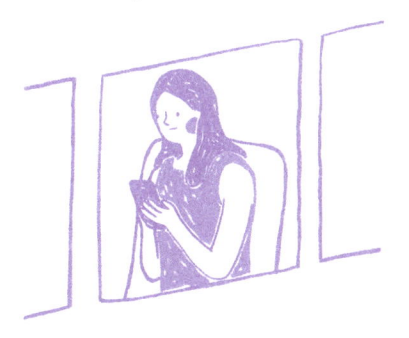

Forgetting – no, even the act of being forgotten – isn't something I seem to have any control over.

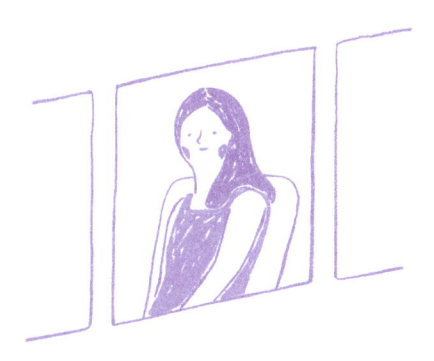

Sometimes, social media features like 'friend suggestions' or 'memories from X years ago' feel more like the pitfalls of the digital and big data era. Sure, they can warm your heart with a wave of nostalgia, but more often, they show up uninvited, pulling unwanted memories into the middle of the day.

Digital relationships often feel light, even disposable. But when you try to cut them off, they're never quite as easy to let go of as they seemed. How much weight should we give to these relationships? When does 'light' become too light? What does it mean to store memories well – and let them go properly? Does hitting the 'block' button really end anything?

I know it's only natural to care about people I once gave my heart to. But even so, there are memories that I still haven't been able to make peace with. So these days, I find myself longing deeply for two things: the right to forget well, and the right to be forgotten gracefully.

12
To Someone I'll Never See Again

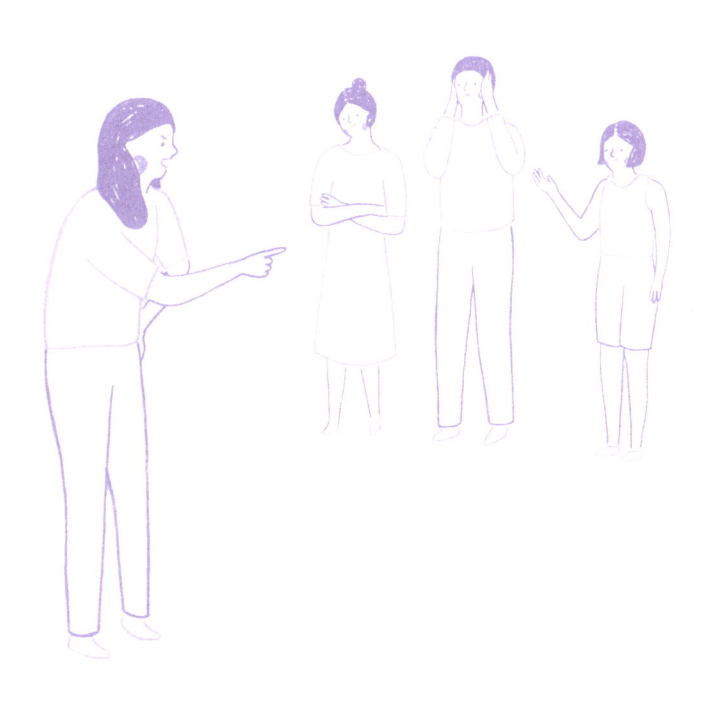

Don't waste energy blaming someone
who'll no longer be in your life.

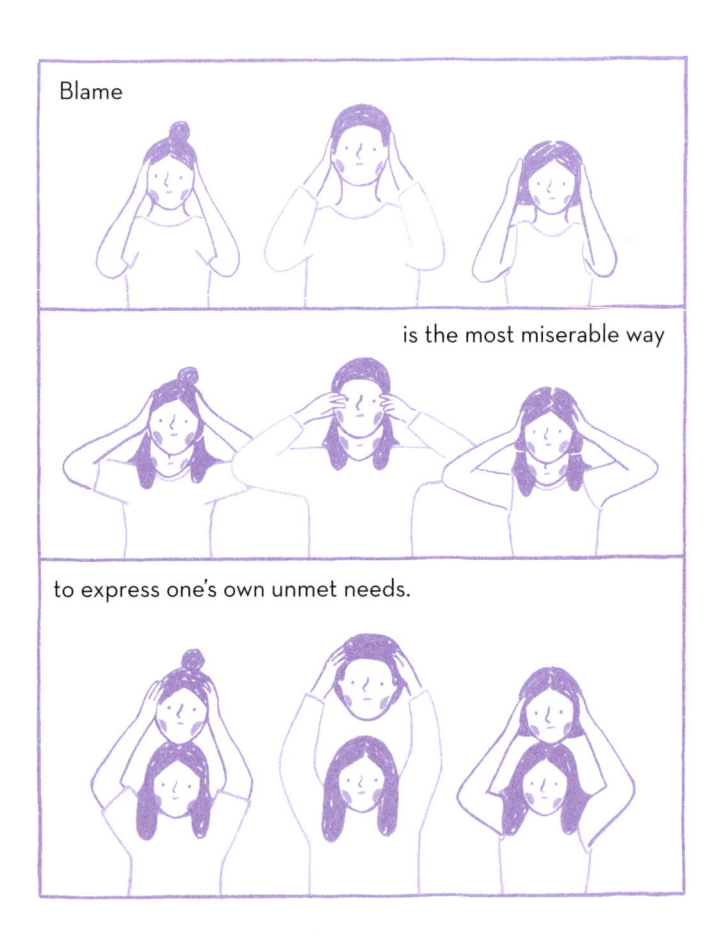

Blame is the most miserable way to express one's own unmet needs.

Hello! I'm the part of yourself you hate, reflected in others.

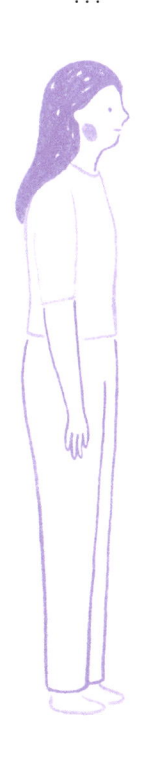

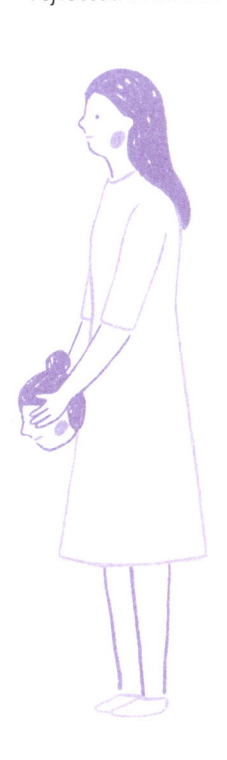

. . .

When I think about my close friends, many of them seem to have personalities completely different from mine. I tend to easily identify myself with others, so I'm often generous toward traits that are different from mine. But I generally find it hard to get along with someone who shares the same flaws I see in myself. So when I get angry at someone, deep down, I'm actually angry at myself.

Negative or antagonistic feelings towards others have a way of circling back and hurting us. Most people blame or lash out at others in an attempt to prove that they are right. The harsher we blame someone, the more we risk giving them a reason to see us as someone who can't even manage their own emotions properly.

Still, if you feel anger rising, take a moment to ask yourself: is this really about them – or is it the flip side of self-blame? Is this person truly worth the cost of your anger, your peace and even your reputation?

Instead of draining ourselves by hating people, why not redirect that energy into giving more love to those who you love? And maybe it's worth pausing before blaming someone you'll never even see again.

13
The 'Relationships Are Hard' Club

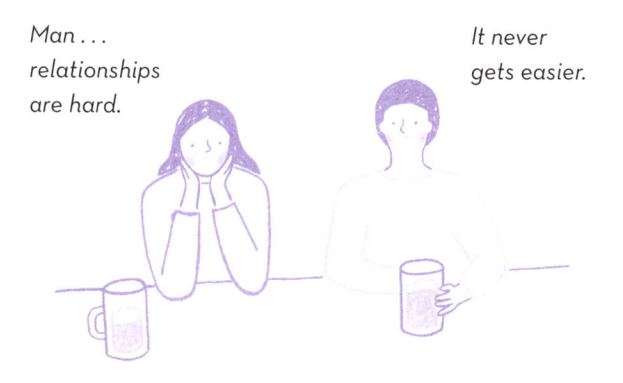

Man... relationships are hard.

It never gets easier.

When you reach that point with someone – where you can openly share that relationships are difficult,

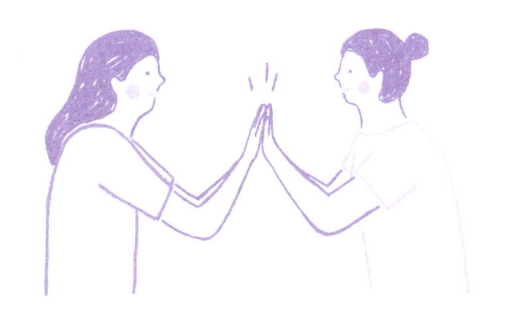

Just between us...

you instinctively feel the connection and click.

[Situationship]

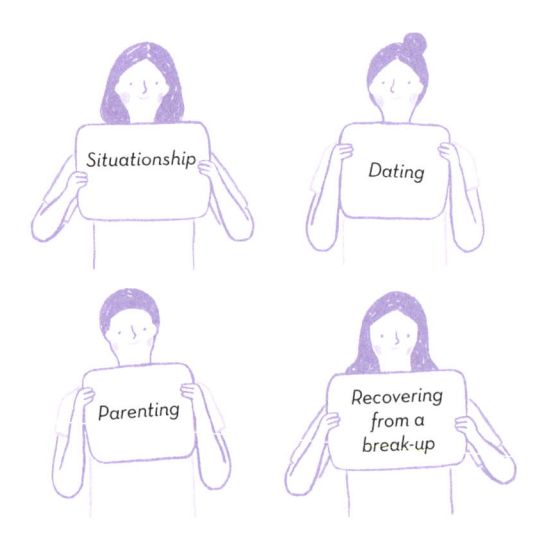

[Dating]

[Parenting]

[Recovering from a break-up]

But as time passes, the connection becomes compartmentalised.

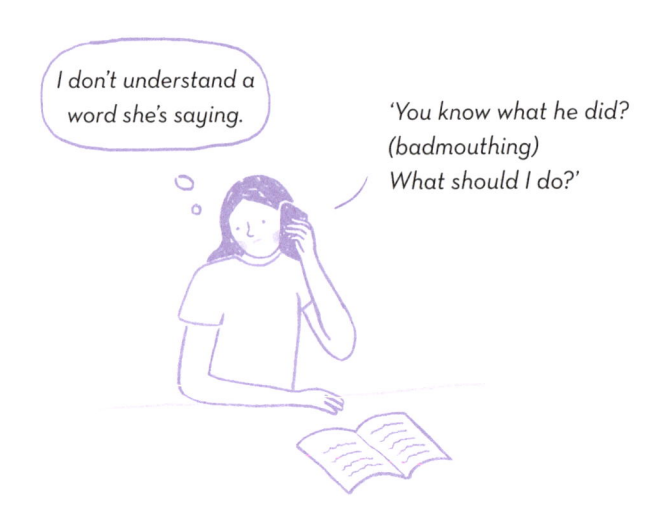

I don't understand a word she's saying.

'You know what he did? (badmouthing) What should I do?'

Sometimes you do not understand them.

Nothing brings people together quite like gossiping about a mutual enemy – especially when they have nothing else in common. Another strong way to bond is through sharing relationship problems. Even the most popular *inssa* or the head of state is bound to have at least one or two issues when it comes to dealing with people.

For me, though, relationship issues are something I rarely talk about – unless it's with someone I deeply trust. Opening up about relationships sends a quiet signal: 'We're close enough now to talk about the messy stuff.'

In fact, sharing these hard conversations shapes bonds that steep like tea – growing richer, closer, and more resonant than other relationships. The only downside is that even the deepest bond can feel shallow again if our personal lives and concerns start to diverge. When our worries no longer overlap, the closeness we built can quietly fade.

Why is it always so hard with people, really? No matter how much we experience them, we only grow more familiar with them, not necessarily better at them. It never truly gets easier.

14
Emotional Hunger

On a sleepless night

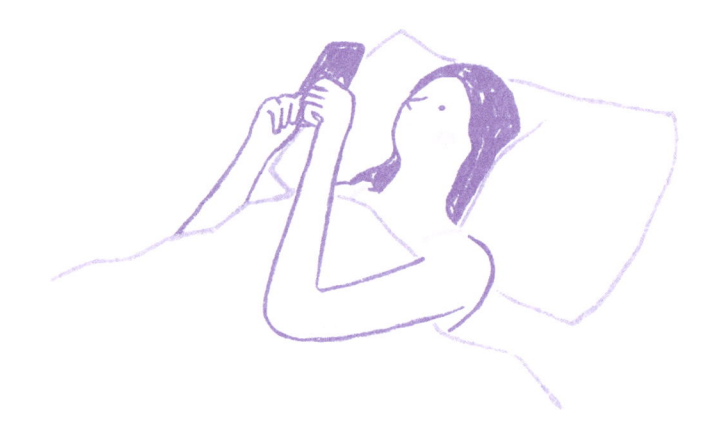

I open the fridge again and again, but nothing seems enough to fill me.

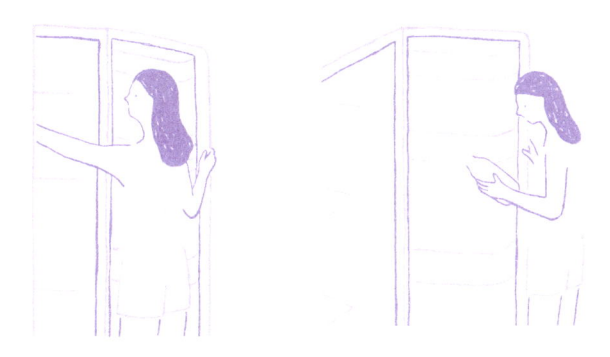

Because what's empty isn't my stomach, it's my heart.

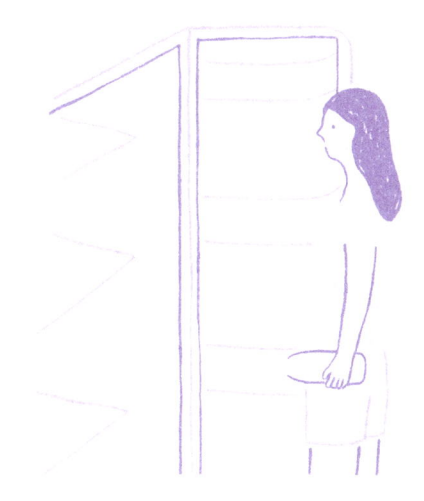

15
Running Into an Old Friend at a Wedding

I vaguely remember the face, but the name just won't come to me.

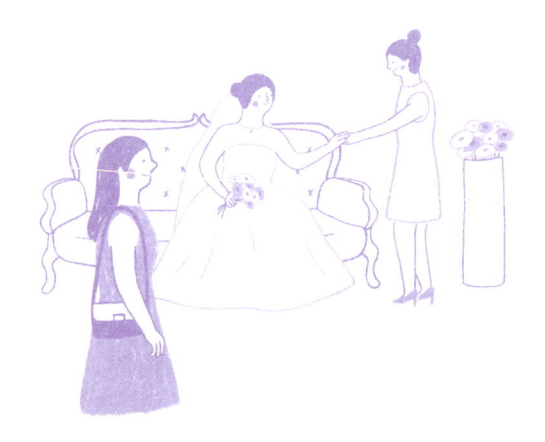

Still, I already smiled and said hello – and now here we are, with nothing to say, awkward silence hanging in the air.

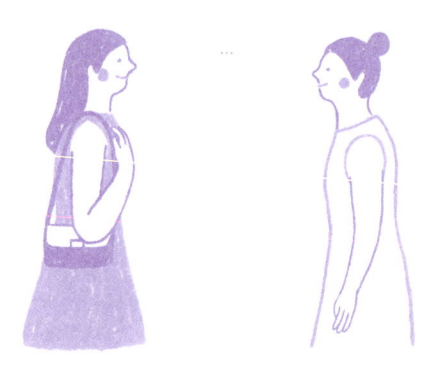

For a moment, I slip back into who I was in school.

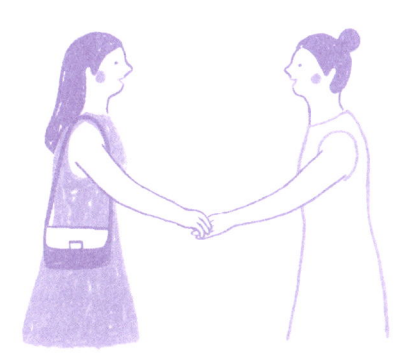

Those were the days. Interesting how different our lives turned out to be.

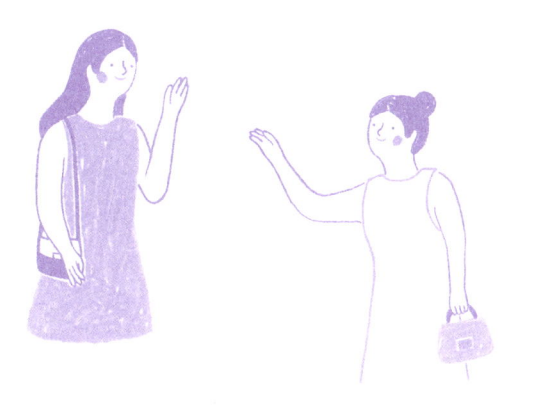

I've never been good at remembering names, so running into an old classmate I haven't kept in touch with is always a little awkward. Out of guilt, I pretend I haven't forgotten, and dig up old memories to fill the silence during our meals.

  Back in school, those cliques felt like the entire world. But after all the highs and lows, seeing how we've each gone on to live our separate lives, I wonder why I once clung so tightly to those small, closed-in relationships. Why did it all feel so serious back then?

  In the end, I couldn't remember their name, and chances are, I'll never see them again after today. So I offer a gentle but fleeting goodbye, then head home, quietly wrapped in a strange, wistful mood.

16
The Opportunity Cost of Excitement

A blind date in December.

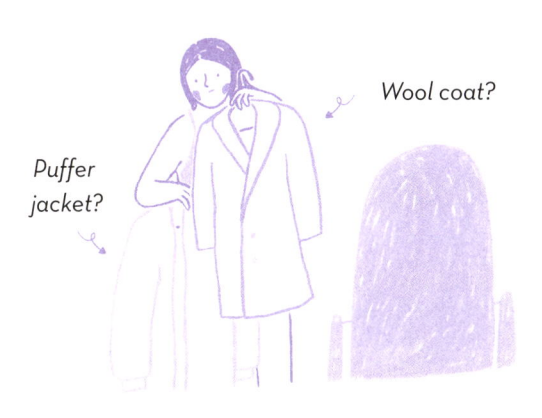

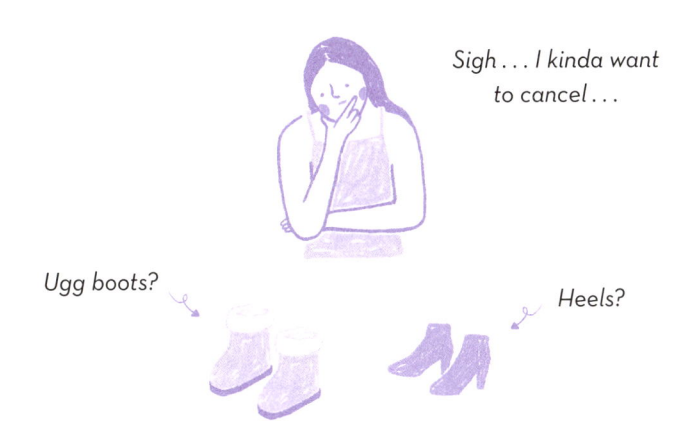

Puffer jacket?

Wool coat?

Sigh . . . I kinda want to cancel . . .

Ugg boots?

Heels?

A date in July.

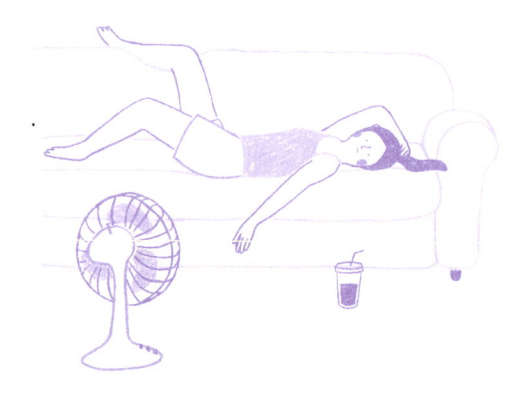

There's always a price for excitement,
which is comfort.

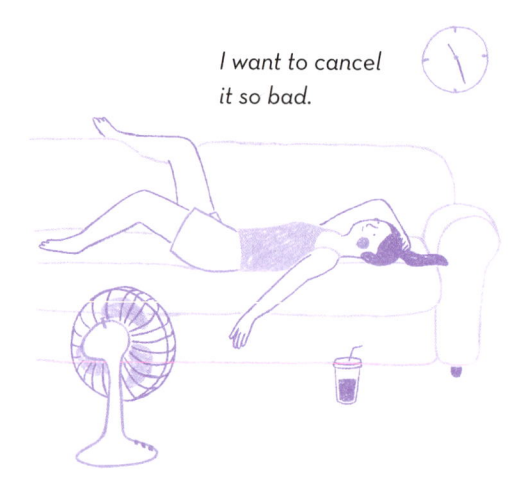

*I want to cancel
it so bad.*

For true homebodies, leaving the house to meet someone in the middle of a hot summer or the dead of winter means true love. Whether on sunny days, rainy days and on all the days in between, their default desire is actively doing 'nothing'.

So, for someone to willingly climb out of a comfy, stretched-out T-shirt and soft fleece pyjamas, and go through the 'getting-ready labour', it takes a level of passion that's worth a few times more than the average person could muster.

Most days, we choose to be alone rather than go through the hassle. And even when we want to feel that spark again . . . ugh, it's just not that easy.

17
I Like the Way Things Are Now

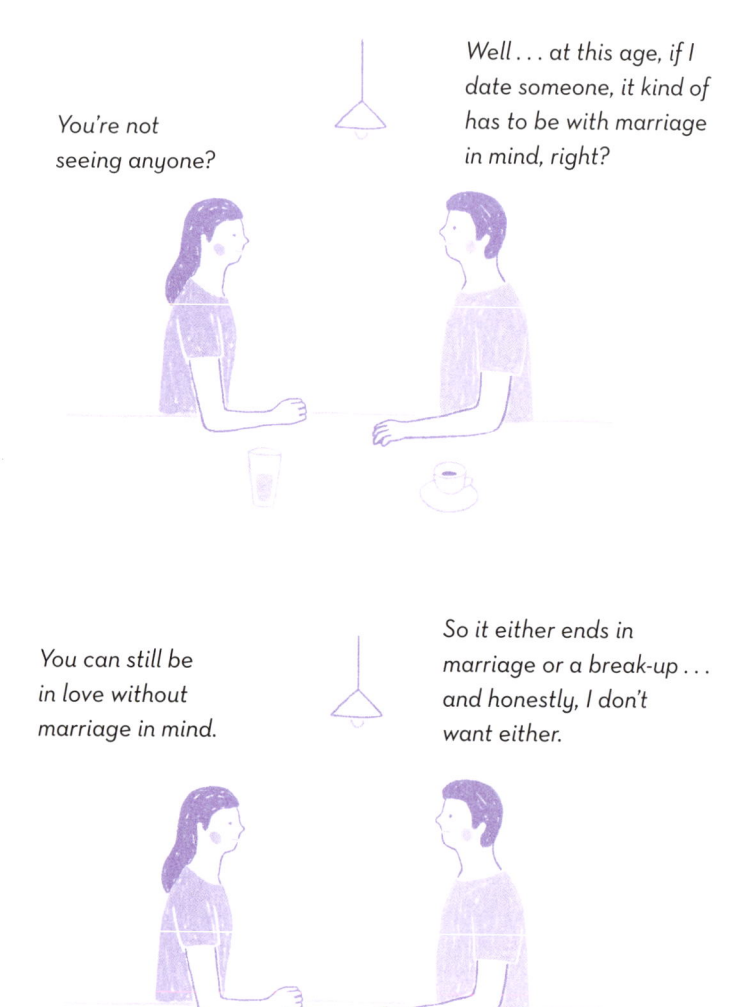

You're not seeing anyone?

Well... at this age, if I date someone, it kind of has to be with marriage in mind, right?

You can still be in love without marriage in mind.

So it either ends in marriage or a break-up... and honestly, I don't want either.

Same. I don't think I'm ready to take care of another life besides my own.

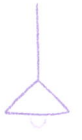

I'm happy with how things are – can we just stay this way?

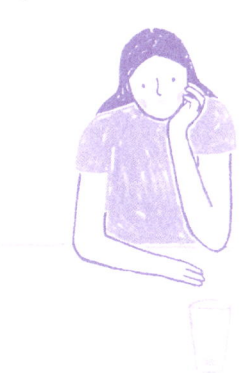

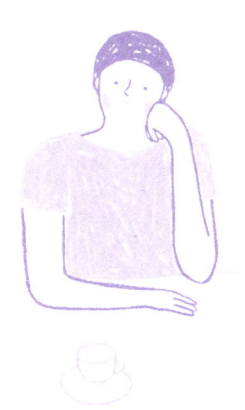

18

The Reason We Slowly Close Our Hearts

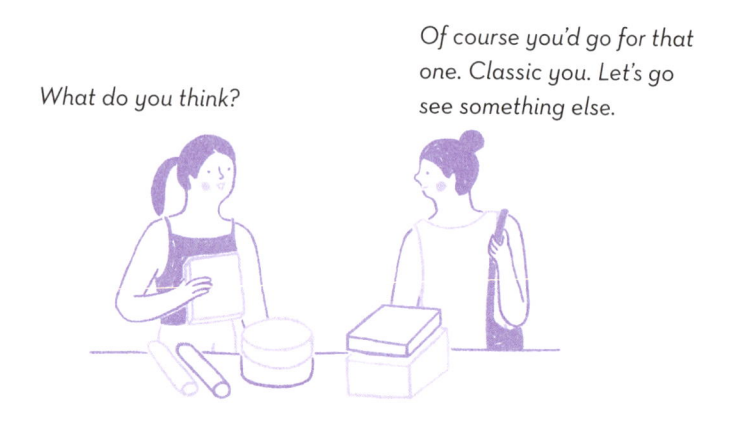

What do you think?

Of course you'd go for that one. Classic you. Let's go see something else.

In a relationship where the smallest preferences and decisions aren't respected,

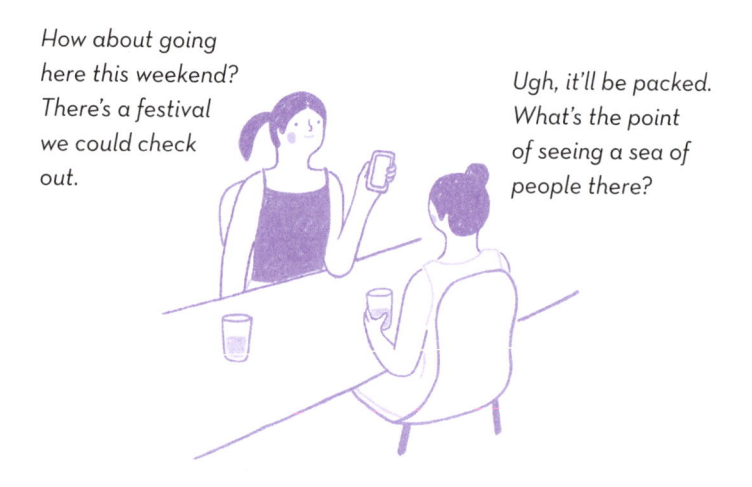

How about going here this weekend? There's a festival we could check out.

Ugh, it'll be packed. What's the point of seeing a sea of people there?

you begin to shut down – quietly, gradually.

I'm thinking of making some YouTube content!

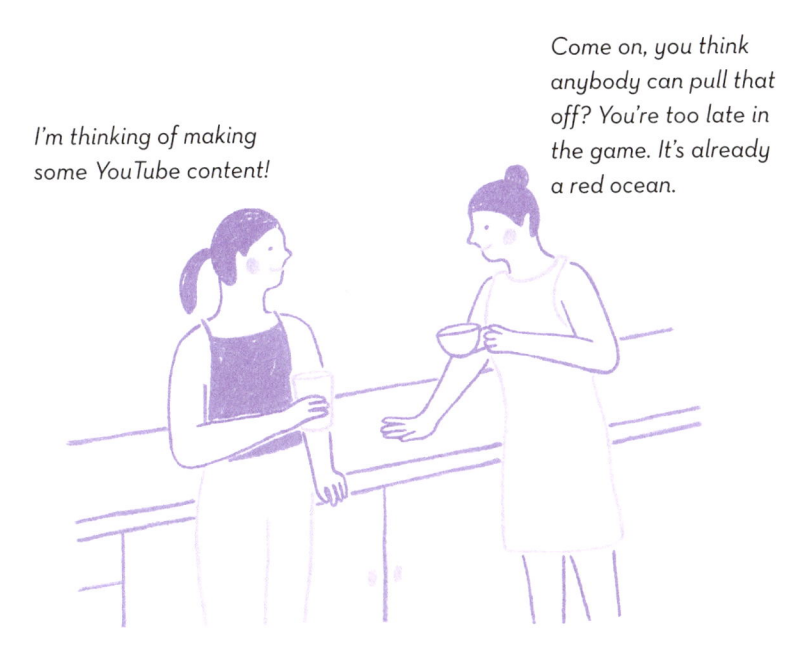

Come on, you think anybody can pull that off? You're too late in the game. It's already a red ocean.

Because those little rejections start to feel like one big rejection of your identity.

So she was always pooh-poohing my ideas!

Oh, come on! What's wrong with her? Just ignore her!

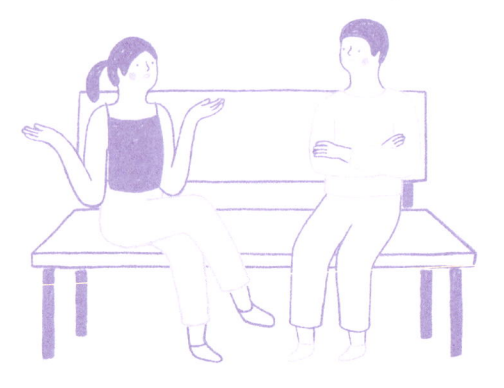

Sometimes, it's enough to respect that they are their decisions to make.

Oh, that's so sweet of you! Seriously, you're the best.

Don't overthink it. What your heart says is the right answer.

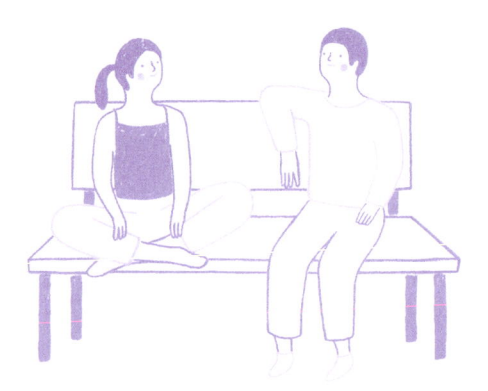

Even if you can't always agree with their decisions.

Maybe because I didn't really go through a so-called rebellious teenage phase, I belatedly had a full-blown second adolescence instead. During that time, I was incredibly stubborn in my relationships. In the face of wounded self-esteem – especially within close relationships – I poured too much energy into trying to prove myself in all the wrong ways. And in doing so, I lost the ability to hear my own voice. Looking back now, it's what I regret the most.

When choices – no matter how small – are repeatedly dismissed, you eventually stop asking yourself what you truly want. Instead, you become consumed with proving your opinion right – not because it matters most, but because you're desperate for it to be acknowledged. It stops being about what feels right for you and becomes about winning. Rejecting the other person's opinion and insisting on your own becomes the only goal.

When that kind of experience continues, trusting your own decisions becomes harder and harder. You start to feel anxious – sometimes overwhelmingly so – even about trying something new or taking the smallest step forwards. Because deep down, you've lost the ability to believe in yourself.

Before challenging someone's opinion, a small gesture of empathy can go a long way. As an American TV series fan, one of my favourite expressions is 'I understand you, but . . .' It's a subtle way of saying, 'You matter to me.' Because sometimes, it's not about agreeing, it's about making the other person feel seen.

MY LITTLE TIPS FOR BALANCING HEALTHY BOUNDARIES IN RELATIONSHIPS

If someone in your life is draining your self-worth and shows no sign of changing, give yourself permission to take some space, at least until you're able to reconnect with what you truly want. Sometimes, what we really need isn't fixing or advice, but quiet respect and heartfelt support.

19
No Break-up is Done Because of Love

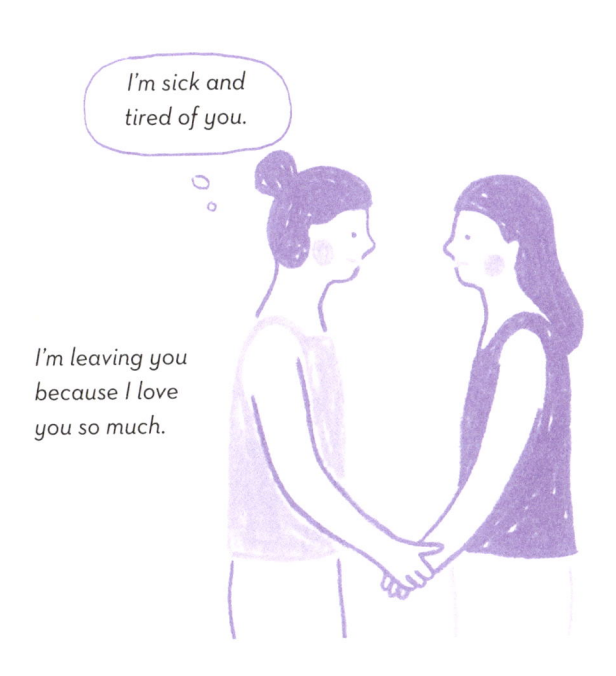

I'm sick and tired of you.

I'm leaving you because I love you so much.

There are a few cunning, misleading words in the world.

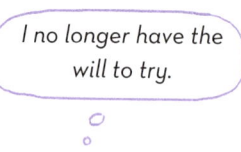

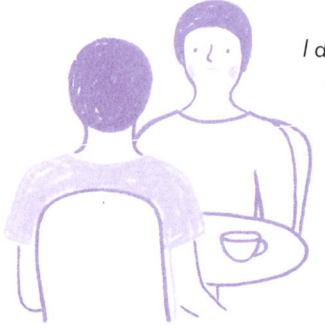

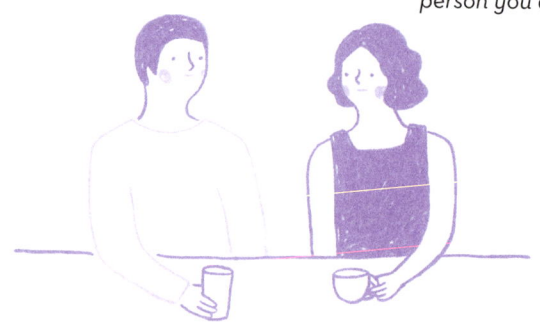

People may break up in spite of love.

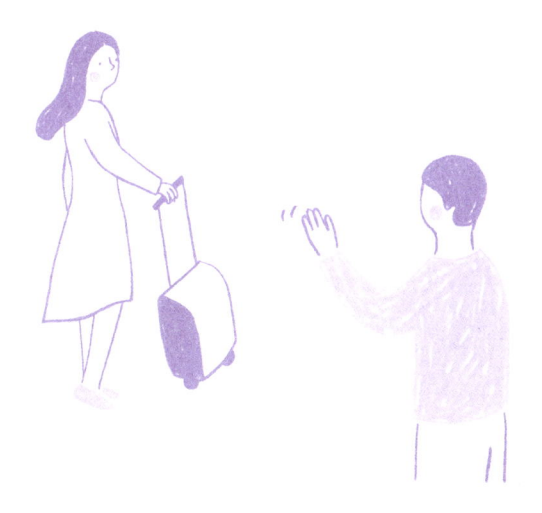

But no one breaks up because they love them
so much. Never.

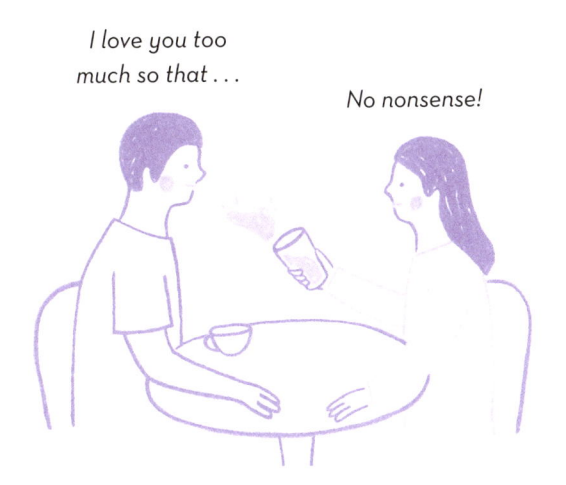

*I love you too
much so that . . .*

No nonsense!

20
Because I Love You So Much

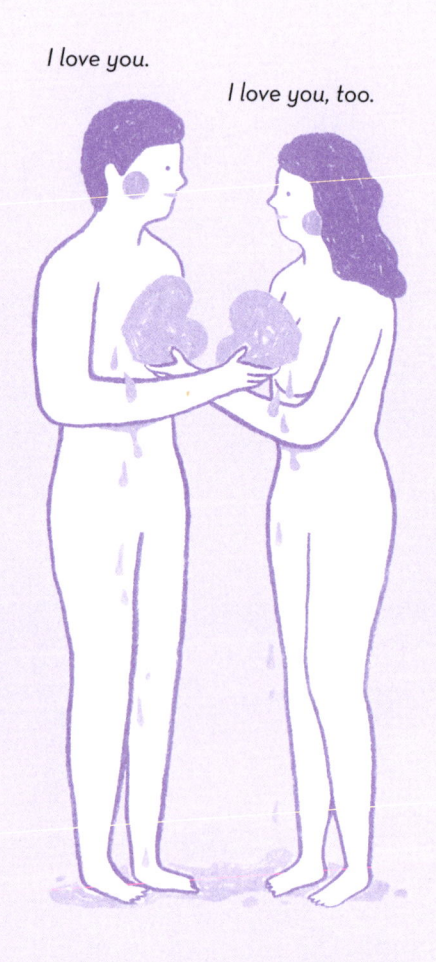

'I'm doing this because I love you so much.' We all know, in our heads, that love should never hurt. But sometimes, despite our best intentions, we end up saying or doing things that leave scars, especially to the ones we love most. The closer we grow to someone, the more we want to know everything about them, to share everything with them. But in that closeness, we sometimes press too hard, and in trying to get close, we hurt them – and then, inevitably, we hurt ourselves.

Even when we regret it, the unkind habits we've grown too used to repeat themselves, as if intimacy is some kind of free pass to say whatever we want, however we want. But if we fill the space between us with emotional impulses and unchecked words, there may no longer be room left for respect – and we may end up losing the person before we lose our so-called 'freedom'.

The sharp point of a heart can sometimes become a blade. So, if someone is hurting you with the excuse, 'It's because I love you,' know this: that is not love. That is violence, hiding behind the mask of love.

MY LITTLE TIPS FOR BALANCING HEALTHY BOUNDARIES IN RELATIONSHIPS

Love and intimacy don't give you permission to say or do whatever you want. No freedom – however personal – should come at the cost of hurting others.

21
Letting the Not Okay Moments Flow By

When buying things

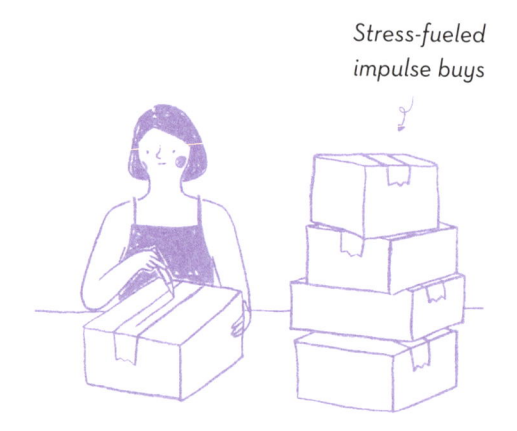

Stress-fueled impulse buys

or eating good food doesn't make me feel better,

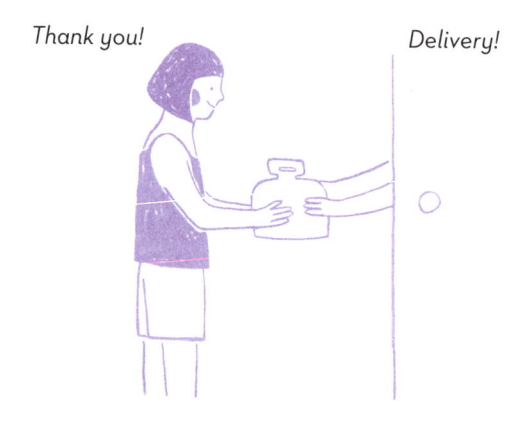

Thank you! *Delivery!*

I honestly don't know what else to do.

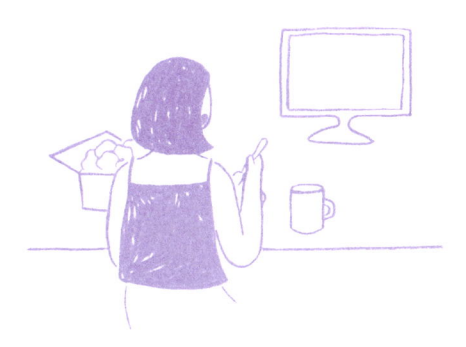

I wish someone could tell me how to become okay again.

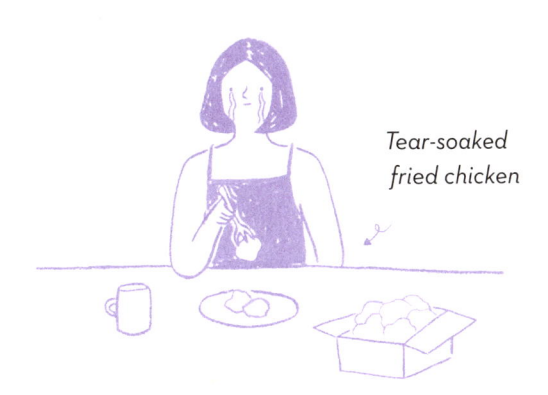

Tear-soaked fried chicken

Anyone who has gone through break-ups knows this: no matter how many times you search online for 'how to deal with heartbreak', you won't find any real solution. You can try to patch up the overflowing grief, hold it back from spilling over. But those are all temporary fixes at best. Your heart teaches you, in the harshest way possible, never to let go of something precious so easily again. Because if you do, you'll be forced to endure this same kind of pain all over again.

It's a cruel truth, but I don't think there's any easy way to recover from heartbreak. You simply have to live through your Not Okay Moments. So far, I haven't found a better way than that.

22
Because I'm Afraid They'll See I'm Not as Cheerful as I Pretend

Some people blend in like air.

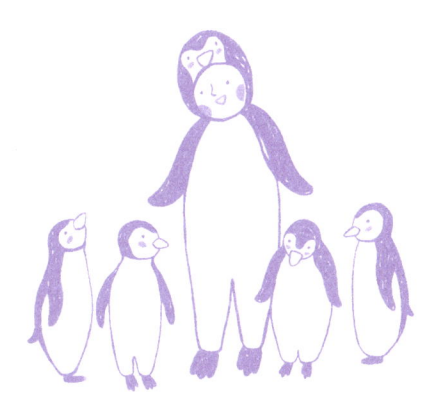

Some feel stressed trying to fit in.

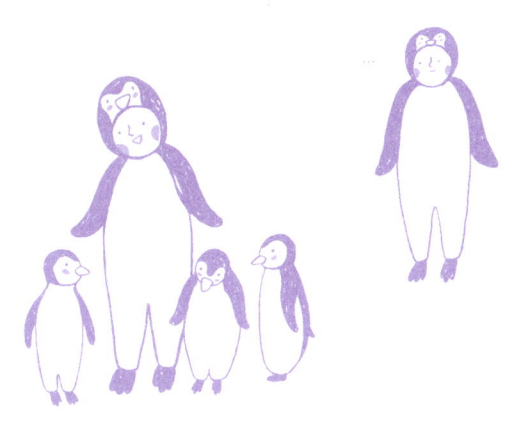

Maybe it's not just me who feels awkward. Maybe they're keeping their distance too.

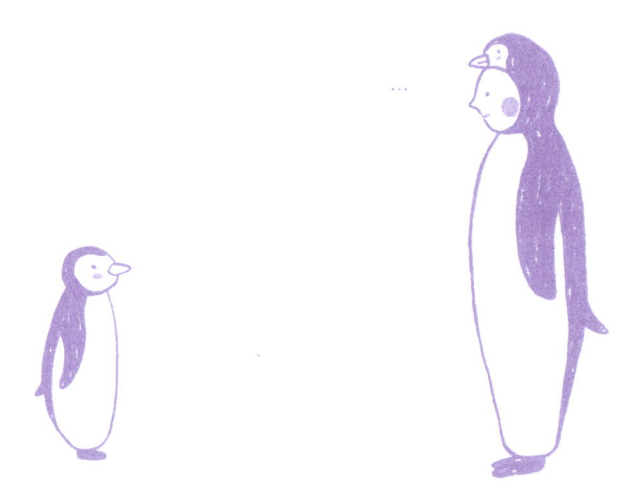

When that happens, don't force it.

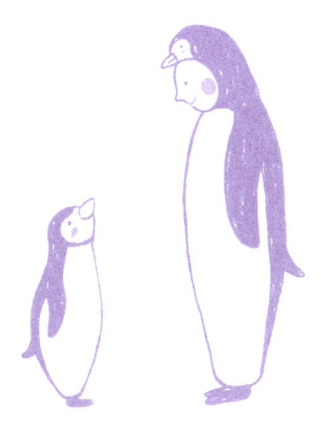

Just take your time, let things be and blend in at your own pace.

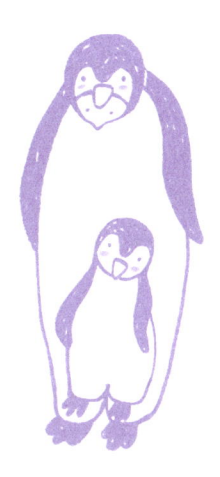

I'm a little shy around new people, but it's not the first meeting that's the hardest for me – it's always the second and third. With people I'll probably never see again, it's not hard to put on a version of myself – the 'me' I'd like them to see. But what's truly uncomfortable is that in-between phase: when you recognise each other's face, but you're not close yet. As time goes on, I start to worry they'll notice that the version of me I showed at first wasn't entirely true, that I'm not always bright. And if they see that, I'm afraid that will drive them away from me.

That kind of worry creates tension, and no matter what I say, it all feels off. And because I'm off and frozen, they find it harder to come to me. If you act out of anxiety and rush to get closer, it often backfires.

When that happens, I'm reminded how much of my attention is still on myself. 'How self-focused must I be to freeze up just at the thought of not appearing perfect?' When I put it in perspective, I realise that most people think about themselves just as much. They're probably just as cautious around me, just as uncertain.

Maybe they're still figuring me out, too. And once I can see that, I begin to notice their heart more clearly.

All we need to do is give each other time to feel safe, to feel seen, to let our guard down at our own pace. And of course, we have to be willing to open a little of our own heart, too.

23
Good Person and Bad Guy

Someone's beloved family

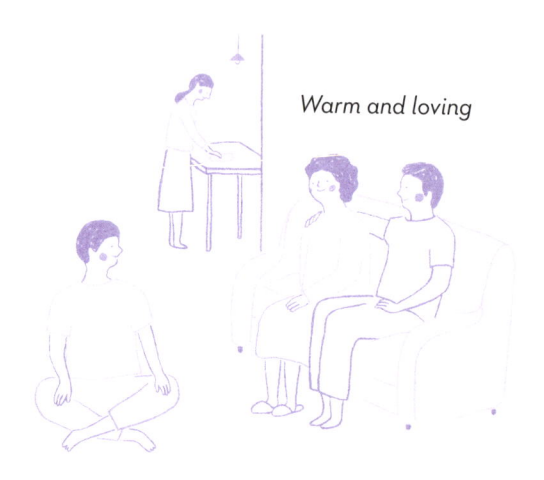

Warm and loving

can be another's nightmare in-laws,

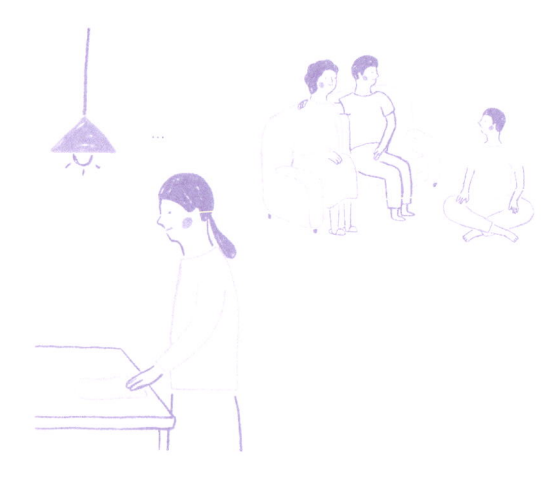

and someone's 'toxic ex' boyfriend

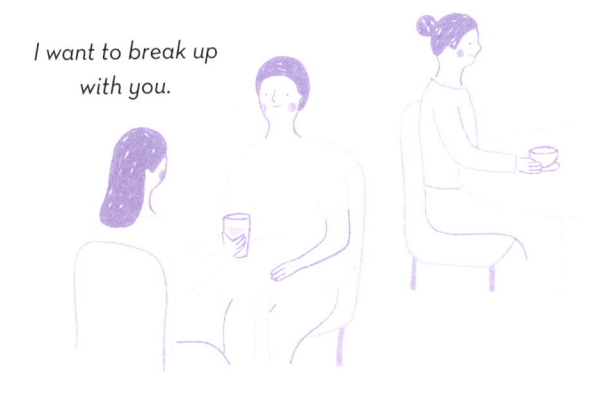

I want to break up with you.

can be someone else's 'Prince Charming' boyfriend.

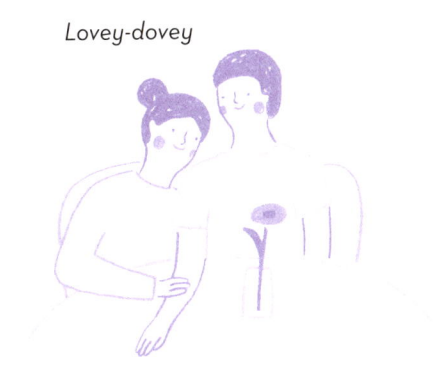

Lovey-dovey

Growing up means learning to see people as more than just one thing.

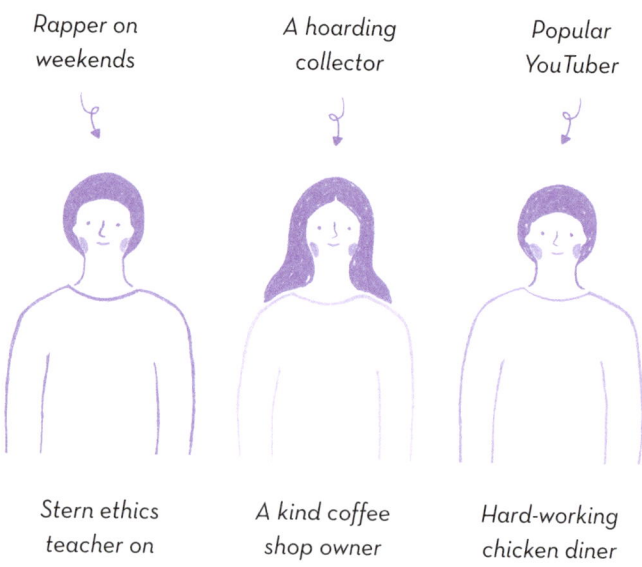

Rapper on weekends	A hoarding collector	Popular YouTuber
Stern ethics teacher on weekdays	A kind coffee shop owner	Hard-working chicken diner deliveryman

Emotions are a strange thing. When I draw for work, I always wish I had a style that's instantly recognisable – a signature look that everyone knows to be mine. But the moment someone says they recognised my art, I get scared. I'm afraid I'll be trapped in a fixed image I can't grow out of. And yet, I often catch myself putting others into the one-dimensional image of the people around me, without even realising it.

It was only as I got older that I realised the woman who had always just been my grandmother was also someone's mother-in-law, and someone's mother. I had to accept, however reluctantly, that a person I had written off completely might be someone else's great love, someone's most romantic story.

The world isn't divided into 'good saints' and 'bad jerks'. And I, too, can't be a good person to everyone I meet. But maybe if I can accept that truth, I'll be able to understand the relationships I never quite could before – with a little more grace.

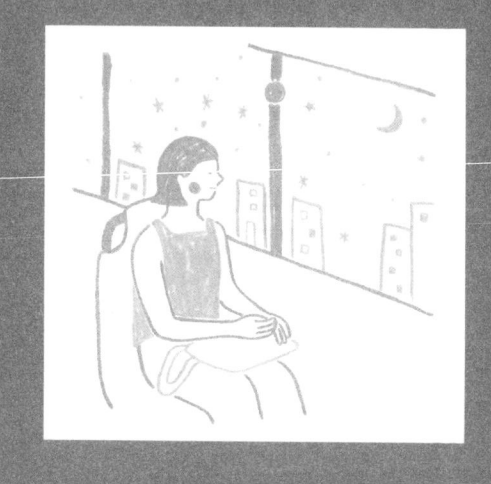

PART 02

IT'S OKAY NOT TO GET ALONG WITH EVERYONE

24
May You Never Be the Lesser in This World

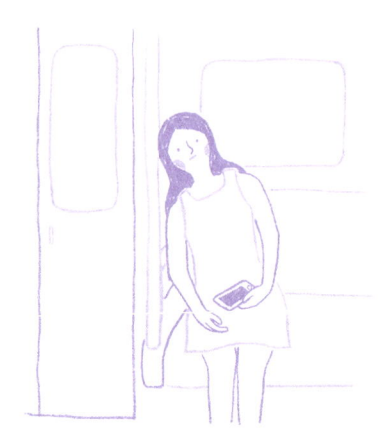

I was always the one who reached out.

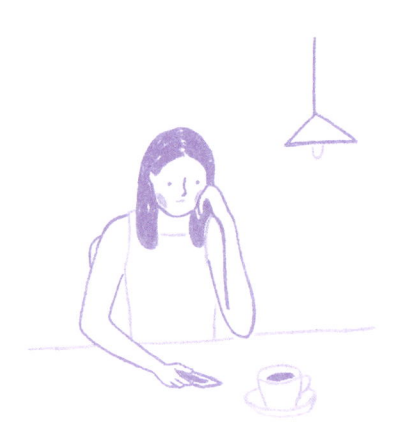

The one who adjusted my time.

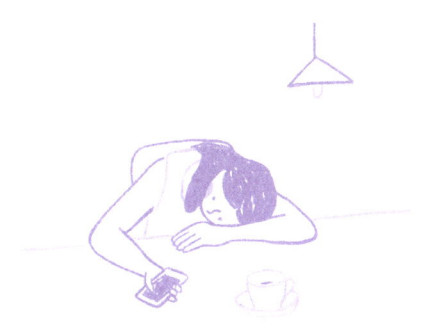

But somehow, I was always sidelined by you.

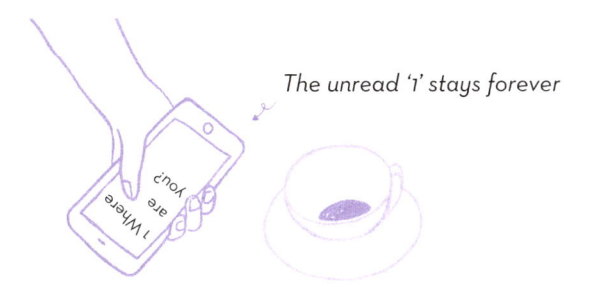

The unread '1' stays forever

From now on, I won't ask anymore

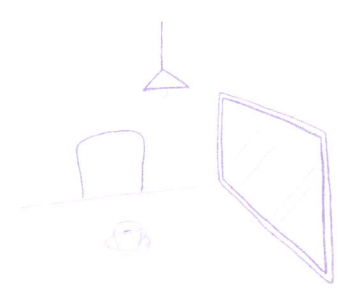

why I was always the one chasing, always second on your list.

I know I don't have to – but in relationships, the one who cares more almost always seems to end up in the lesser position. Not just in love, but even in friendships, acquaintanceships and with colleagues – you can sometimes sense a subtle difference in how much each person cares.

Do you ever find yourself over-interpreting small acts of kindness or quietly stewing over someone else's indifference? If it happens often, chances are you've placed yourself in the 'lesser' role in that relationship.

When the circle of people in your life grows smaller, loneliness can feel sharper.

And when you find yourself needing people too much, you might start feeling grateful just for their presence, as if their existence alone is a gift.

Of course, everyone expresses care in different ways. But if someone always puts themselves first in the relationship, you don't need to feel grateful just for being kept around.

Relationships are meant to be give and take, after all. They're not favours. The other person also gains something from knowing you – you don't owe them just because they showed up.

The roles shift naturally over time. Even if I never intended it, there were times when I might have been in a position of power over someone, or perhaps I still am without realising it. That's why I don't need to pity myself too much for the times when I was, or still am, the one with less power.

But if you currently find yourself taking on that role, remember this: that attitude can carry over into future relationships, and even into your relationship with yourself. And if you never step out of the 'lesser' role, you might slowly start becoming the lesser one not just in one relationship – but to the world itself.

25
Uncomfortable Means Uncomfortable

When you call out somebody for being rude to you,

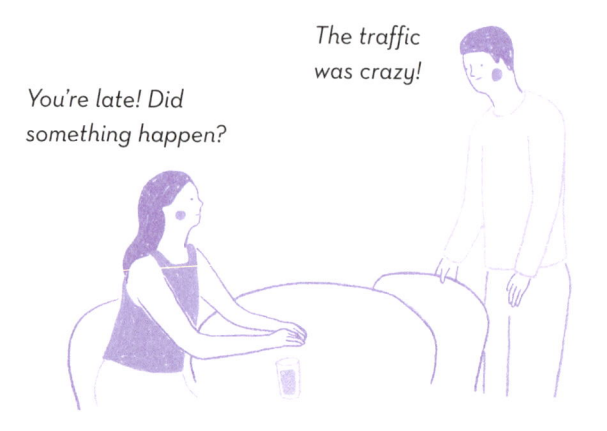

You're late! Did something happen?

The traffic was crazy!

when the other person doesn't seem sorry at all,

You could've just told me you'd be late!

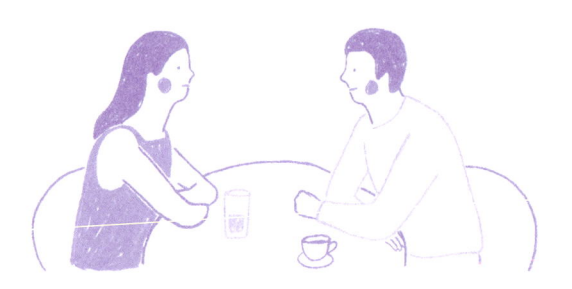

you feel as though you're the bad person.

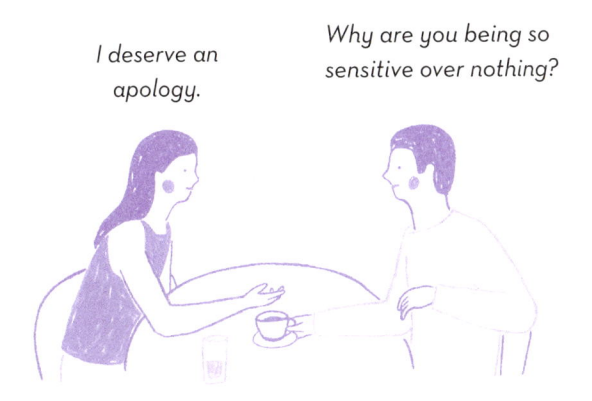

I deserve an apology.

Why are you being so sensitive over nothing?

When actually, they were the one who crossed the line.

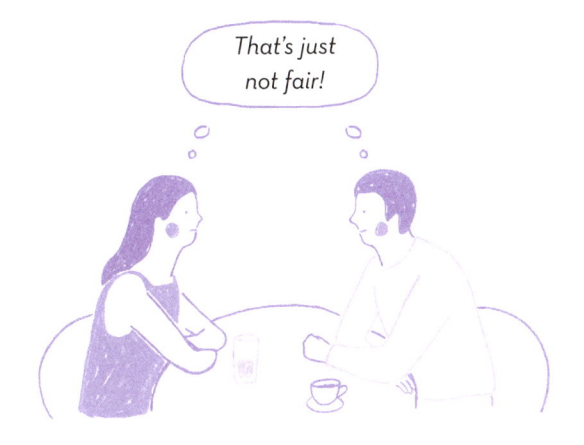

That's just not fair!

Some people have a strange talent for deflecting blame; when I point out their wrongs, they twist the situation until I'm the one feeling guilty. They slap labels on my reactions to be too sensitive or overreacting. And even though I know in my head that I'm not the one at fault, my heart shrinks and I start to doubt myself. So I began asking others: 'This happened, and it made me feel uncomfortable. Am I being too sensitive?' Then I spiral - wasting my life imagining how someone else might have reacted if they were in my shoes.

But at the end of the day, if I feel uncomfortable, then it is uncomfortable. My feelings don't need to be validated by others to be true. In a world full of opinions and overreach, I hope we can at least grant our own feelings the freedom to exist - just as they are.

MY LITTLE TIPS FOR BALANCING HEALTHY BOUNDARIES IN RELATIONSHIPS

My relatively sensitive nature should never be used as a reason to dismiss what I feel. If you ever find yourself being in discomfort, remind yourself: 'If I feel uncomfortable, then it is uncomfortable.'

26
To Console Free from Comparison, to Celebrate Free from Anxiety

Behind the comfort I offer you in your struggle,

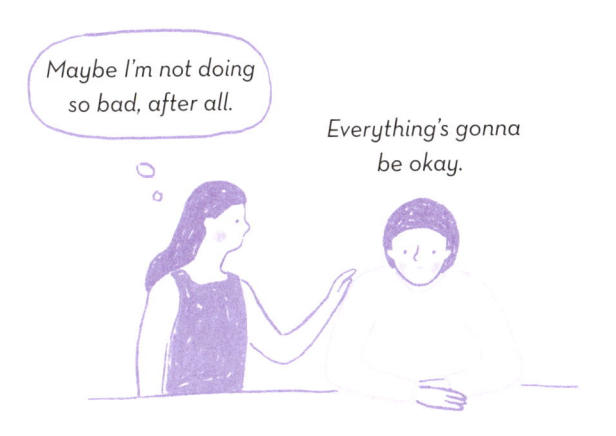

Maybe I'm not doing so bad, after all.

Everything's gonna be okay.

behind the sincere encouragement, I flinch at the chill of my own heart.

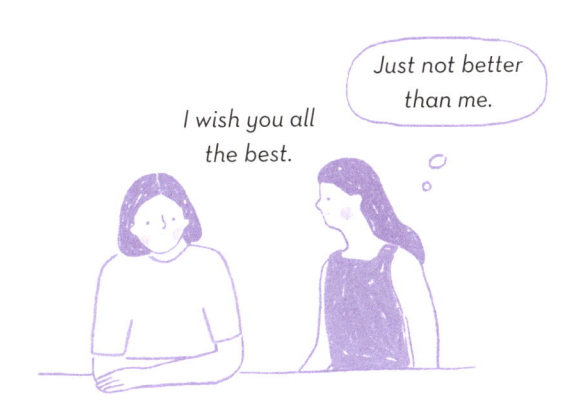

I wish you all the best.

Just not better than me.

I was left feeling disappointed in myself.

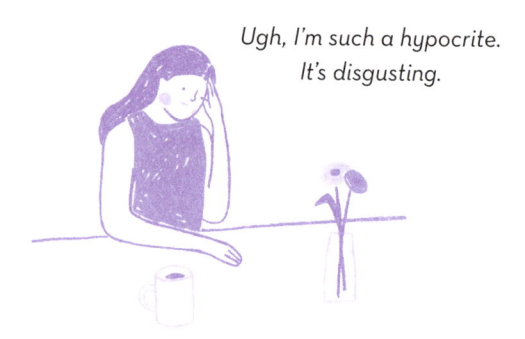

Ugh, I'm such a hypocrite. It's disgusting.

The hollow comfort or lingering anxiety from comparing myself to others.

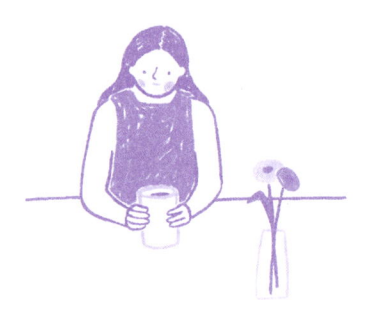

Dear heart, when did you grow so hardened?

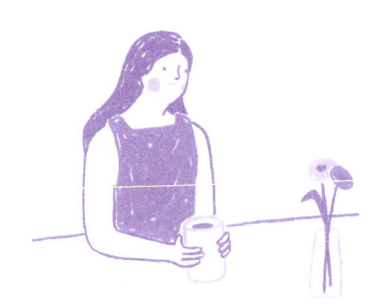

I often get disappointed in myself when I fail to truly comfort or celebrate others. When I offer sympathy to their suffering, at the same time, a part of me feels secretly relieved that I'm not the one going through it. I congratulate a friend's success, but something in me shrinks inside.

In striving to fulfil the duties of adulthood and chasing reassurance by keeping myself in check, had I, without even knowing it, become used to measuring myself against the world's endless comparisons?

Had my heart grown harsher, gripped by the fear that unless I pushed someone else aside to climb higher, my own existence would be at risk? The most dangerous thing about comparison is that it becomes a habit. It becomes second nature, regardless of how much you're already accomplishing. But true self-confidence doesn't come from being ahead of others – it comes from embracing who you are, objectively and without judgement. And once you remember that, you begin to offer people you love the kind of comfort that doesn't need comparison, the kind of congratulations that's free from anxiety.

27
An Eye for an Eye, a Person for a Person

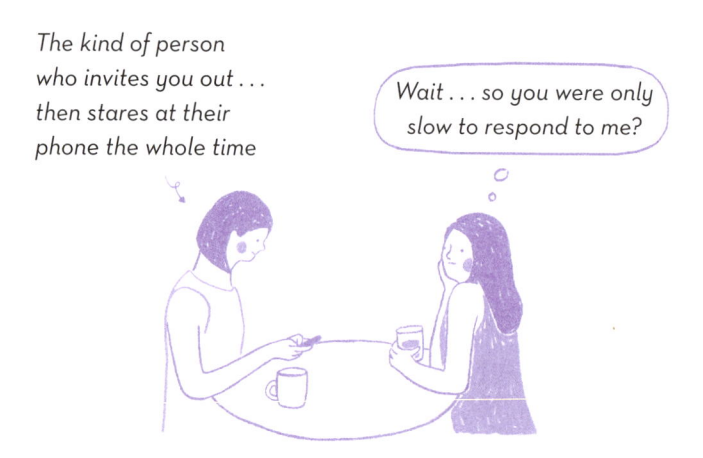

The kind of person who invites you out... then stares at their phone the whole time

Wait... so you were only slow to respond to me?

To someone who is rude to me ➔ I don't have to be rude back, but I don't owe them kindness either.

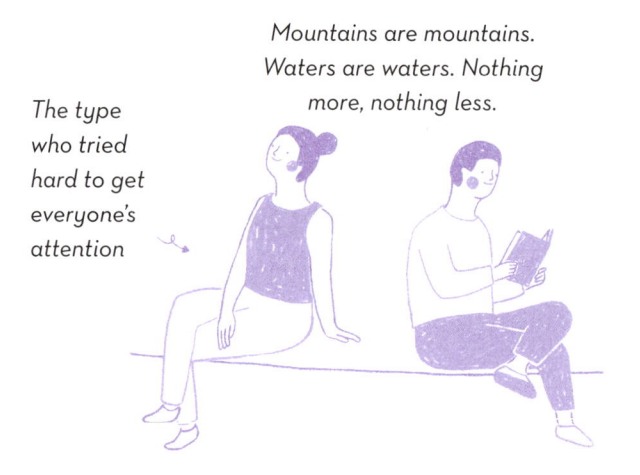

The type who tried hard to get everyone's attention

Mountains are mountains. Waters are waters. Nothing more, nothing less.

To someone who doesn't care about me ➔ there's no reason for me to care about them.

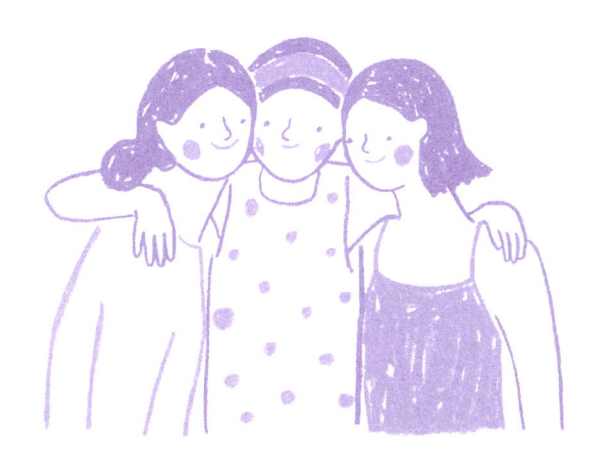

The kind of person who treats me well ➔
treat them well back.

28
Between Stability and Passion

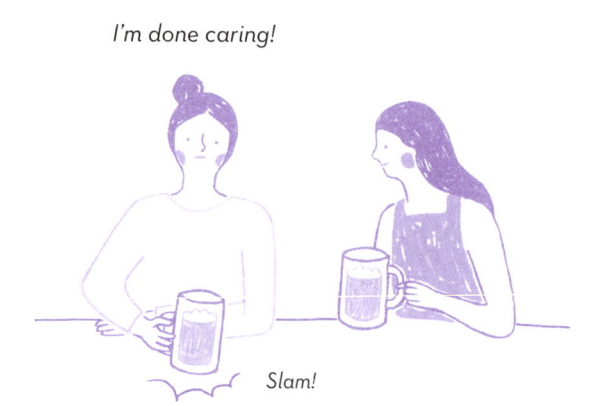

I'm done caring!

Slam!

I just want someone steady and comfortable to be with.

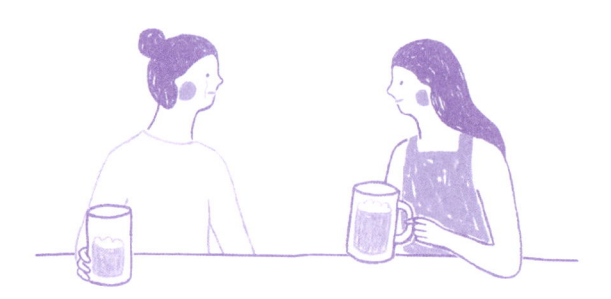

But we know that part of us ... still longs for ...

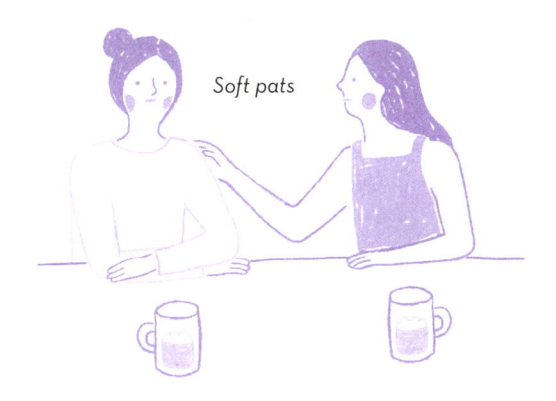

Soft pats

fire.

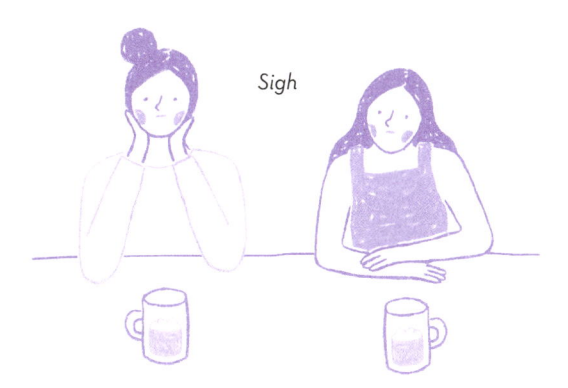

Sigh

I once heard a line from a TV show: 'Romance feels like an adult version of dreaming about what's ahead.' Something that gives you a reason to look forward to tomorrow. What we prioritise in a romantic relationship – emotional safety, joy, connection – varies from person to person, but if there's one thing we all want, it would be fun. Yes, we fall in love because we want it to be fun. No matter how warm, kind or dependable someone is, if it's not fun to be around them – if there's no shared laughter, not even a matching sense of humour – romance probably won't bloom.

But here's the problem: another name for fun and excitement is instability, and on the flip side, security often comes with boredom. You can't have both. You can't feel utterly safe and endlessly thrilled at the same time. It's like a client asking for a design that's both minimal and glamorous. It just doesn't work like that.

Maybe that's why I've never met someone who feels like a 'perfect match'. However, perhaps it's not that the right person doesn't exist – maybe it's just that people who balance both extremes are rare to find, to begin with. If you want stability, you have to accept a little stillness. If you can't give up the thrill, you have to be open to a little chaos. Or at the very least, you should know how much instability you can live with. Before we get into relationships, maybe we should take a moment to ask ourselves one simple question: What are the values I absolutely cannot give up on?

29
It's Okay to Be Uncool

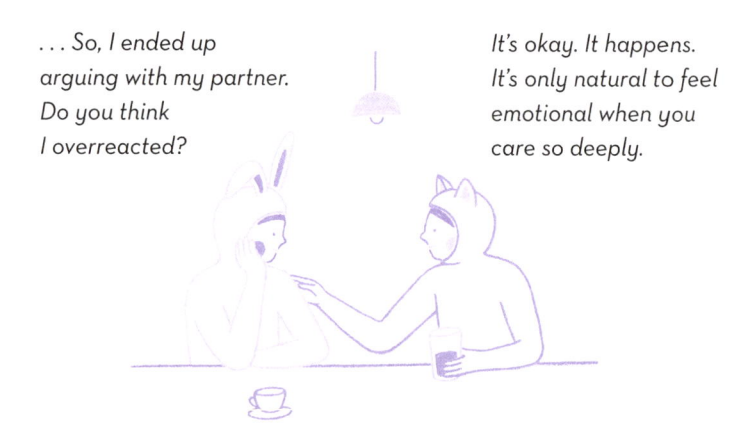

... So, I ended up arguing with my partner. Do you think I overreacted?

It's okay. It happens. It's only natural to feel emotional when you care so deeply.

When you're in love, don't be too hard on yourself for being unreasonable.

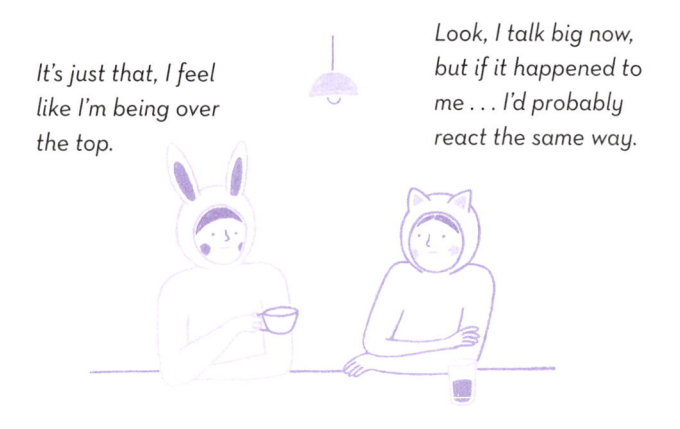

It's just that, I feel like I'm being over the top.

Look, I talk big now, but if it happened to me ... I'd probably react the same way.

Love, by nature, is never entirely reasonable.

See ya

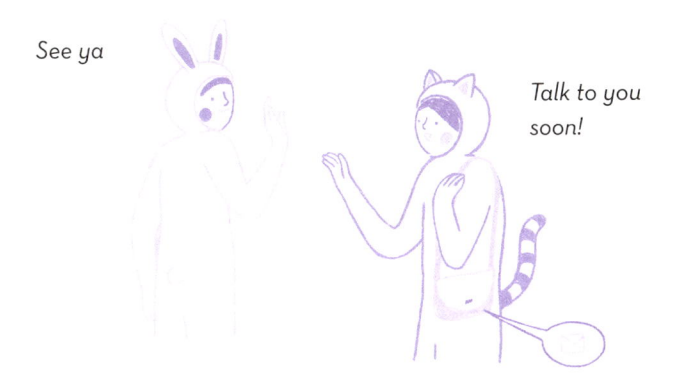

Talk to you soon!

We just don't talk about the messy parts.

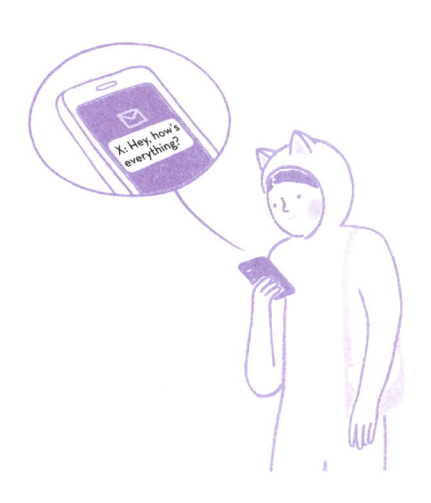

The truth is, there's no such thing as a 'cool' relationship or a 'cool' break-up.

30
To the Worrier Who Worries About Worrying

I know the thrill of liking someone is enough
on its own – but still, fear finds a way in.

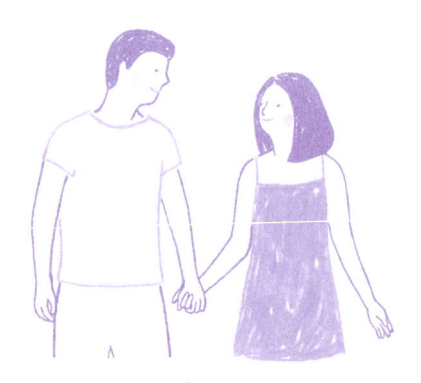

The fear that I'm falling for you, and you're not for me.

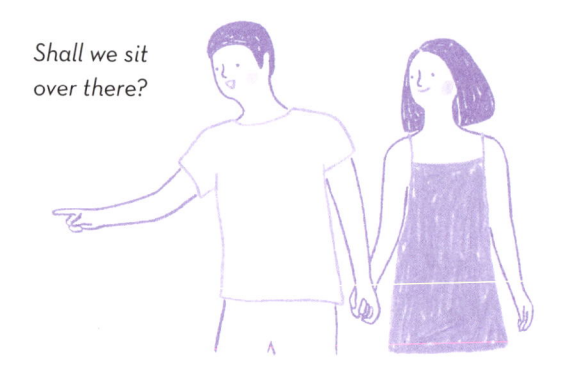

Shall we sit over there?

When all I wanted was casually seeing you,
nothing complicated.

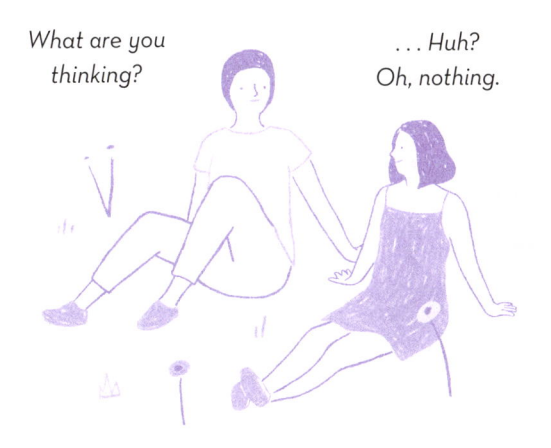

What are you thinking?

... Huh? Oh, nothing.

Yet, somewhere deep down, I'm already thinking it
might hurt less if I hold a little of myself back.

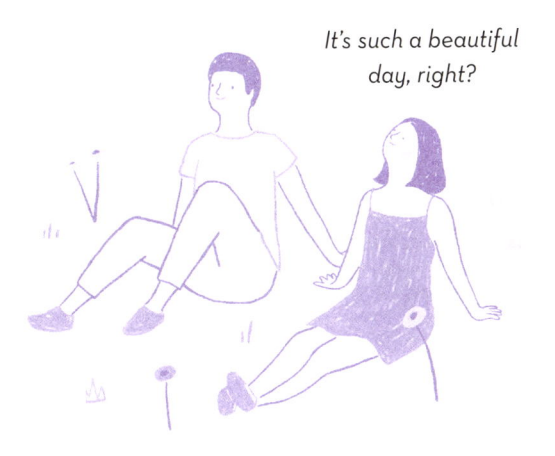

It's such a beautiful day, right?

There's something I hope people who worry about everything, especially when it comes to new relationships, can remember. No matter how much you try to predict the future, imagining the worst won't actually protect you from getting hurt. If anything, that anxiety might lead you to overreact, to push too hard or to act out of fear before anything has even gone wrong – and that can be what ends up hurting the relationship.

Of course, I'm not saying you should throw your heart wide open recklessly, like a child with no sense of boundaries. There's strength in protecting your heart and choosing when – and how much – to let someone in. That window is entirely up to you.

Still, I hope your fear of the future doesn't rob you of the little, precious moments in the present. It's okay to gently push those worries aside for now.

> **MY LITTLE TIPS FOR BALANCING HEALTHY BOUNDARIES IN RELATIONSHIPS**
>
> It's never too late to worry – when there's actually something to worry about. Don't let fear take over for things that haven't even happened yet.

31
When It Doesn't Go Your Way, Go Your Heart's Way

Why is it that my heart never listens to me?

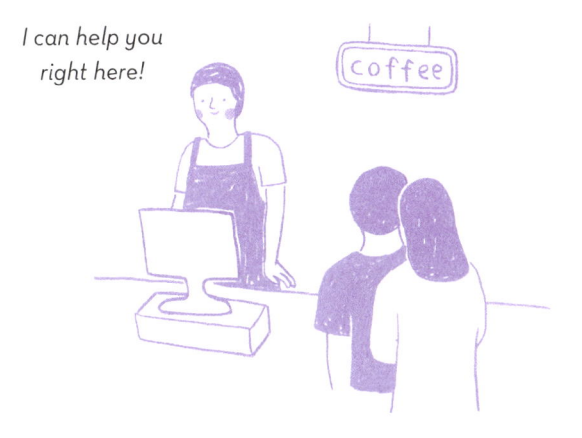

I can help you right here!

coffee

Sometimes, feelings appear out of nowhere, even when I'm not looking for them.

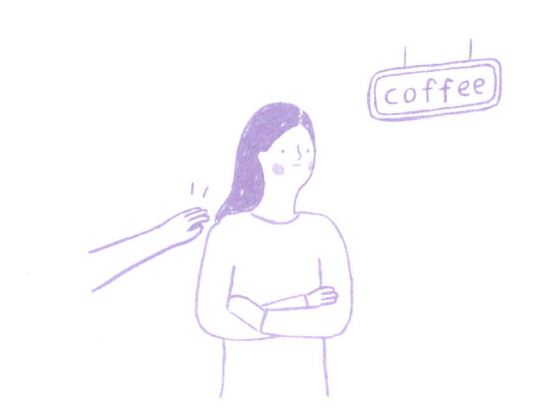

coffee

And other times, feelings I held onto so tightly simply disappear.

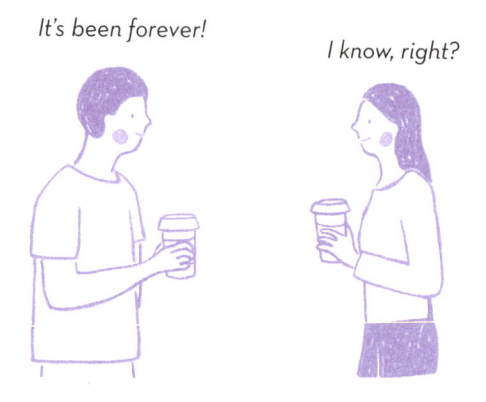

It's been forever!

I know, right?

Maybe, sometimes, the best thing we can do is stop resisting and simply go with the flow.

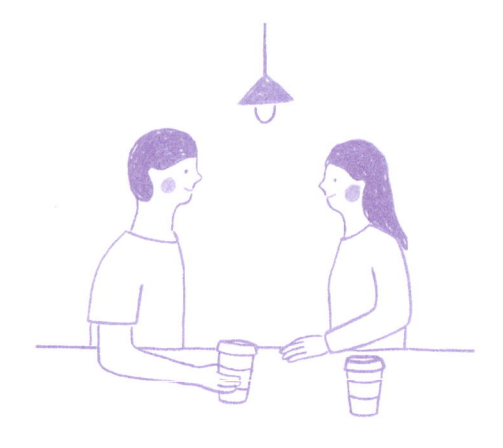

32
Dry Comfort Over Forced Forgiveness

One way to face the pain of being hurt by someone without letting it break you

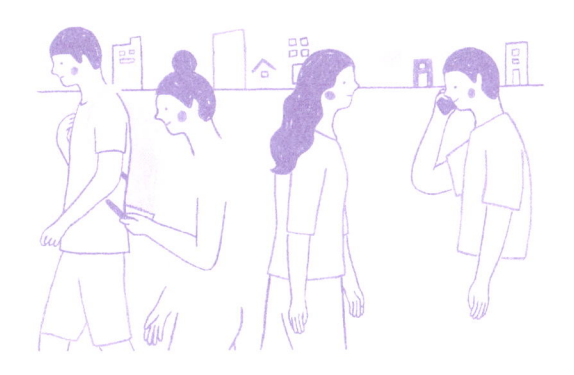

is to dull your senses just a little, and look at it with a dry, quiet gaze.

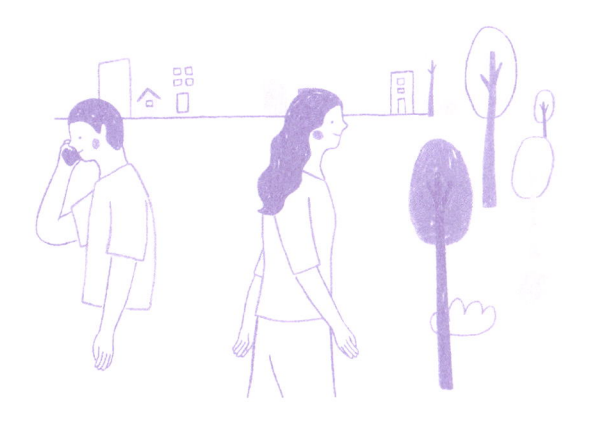

Not with forced forgiveness, or with exaggerated empathy.

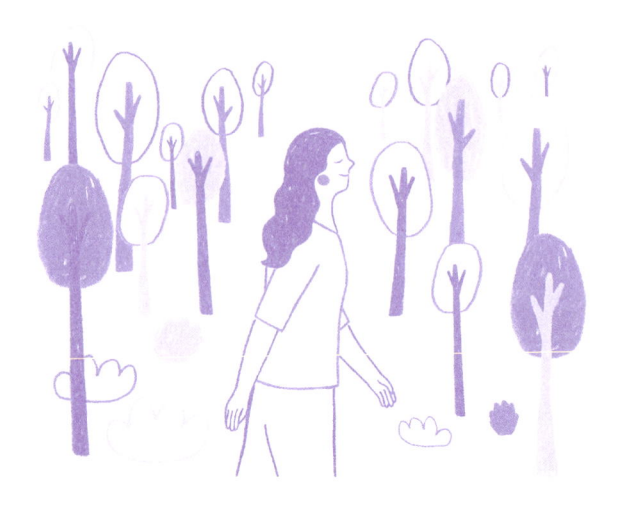

But simply by acknowledging what happened exactly as it is.

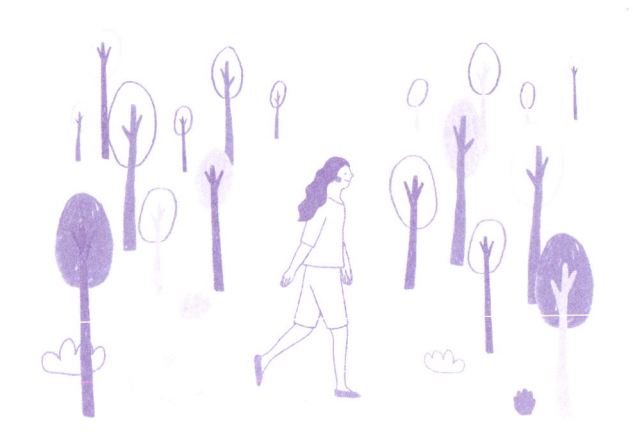

It's a small but special way to comfort myself.

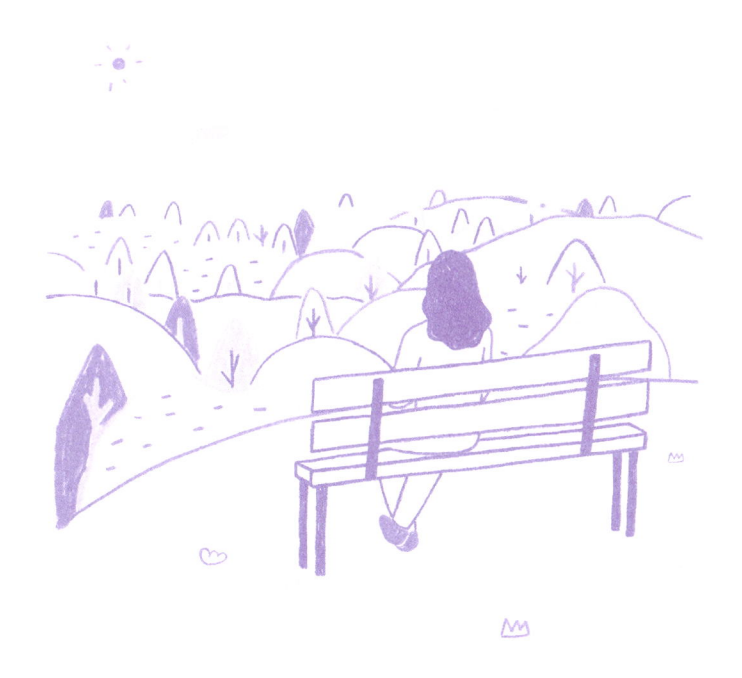

Every time I get hurt by someone, my mind tries to brush it off – but a certain amount of pain always seeps into my senses and settles in my heart, becoming a part of who I am now. When I read to soothe those emotional wounds, I don't reach for fiction or essays but psychology or self-help books. It helps to see people's actions through the lens of evolution or behavioural science – to shift the weight of pain into something more abstract, something I can look at without drowning in it.

Betrayal, break-ups, emotional and physical trauma – the pain these relationships leave behind can be sharp, but what often hurts more is not being able to accept the fact that they did something 'I would never do'.

We don't need to revisit those memories every time they resurface. But if a wound begins to block your growth, maybe it's time to face it – just once – and move through it. And if that feels too painful, then take a colder, more clinical approach: look at the memory from a distance. This isn't about straining all my generosity to forgive the person who hurt me, or about granting them a pardon I don't truly mean. It's about seeing them as if from a third-party perspective, removing any link to myself. It's closer to understanding, at least intellectually, by seeing them not as 'the person who hurt me,' but simply as 'a flawed human being.' And when you've done that, when the memory has been reframed and digested, you may finally find the pain loosening its grip.

33
All the Emotions You Feel are Always Right

The sound I love the most.

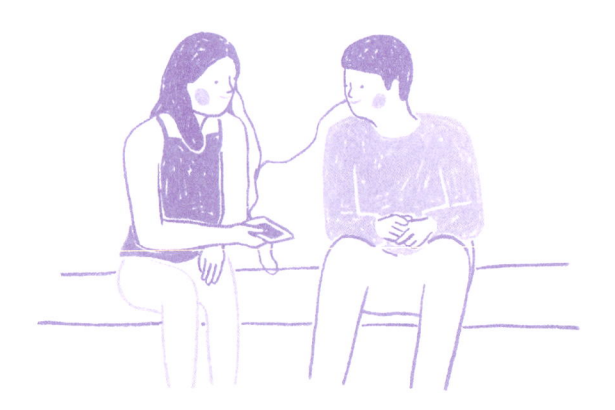

The sound I never want to hear again.

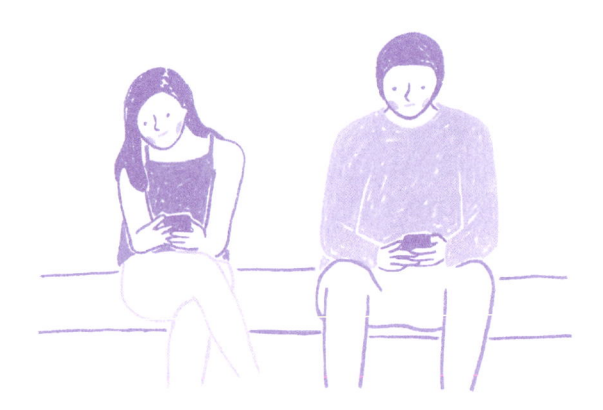

The voice I know too well.

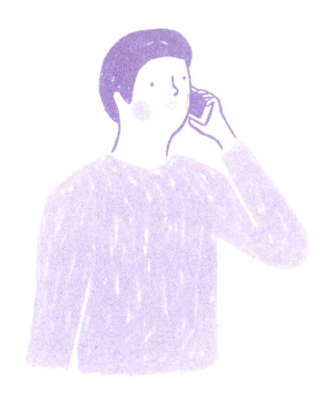

The voice I wish I could forget.

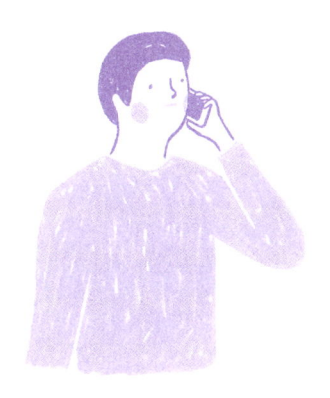

The scent I love the most.

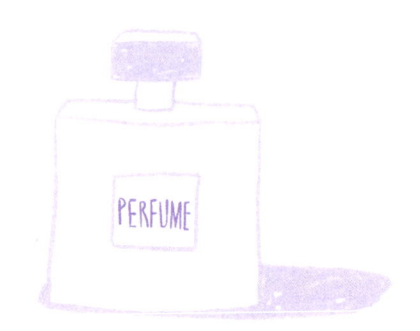

The scent I hate the most.

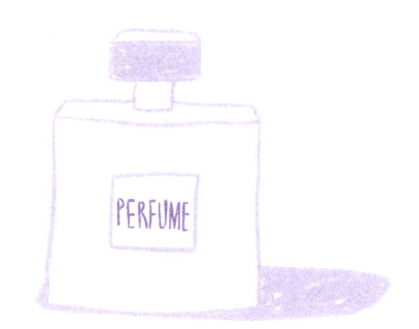

I like that about you.

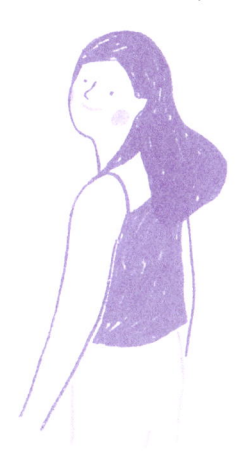

I hated that about you.

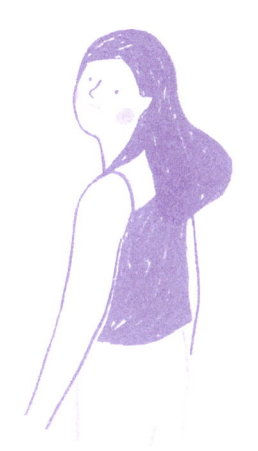

We are always meant to be.

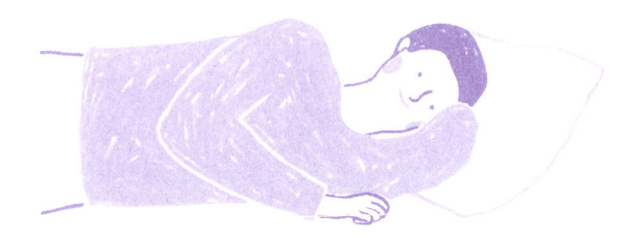

We were never meant to be.

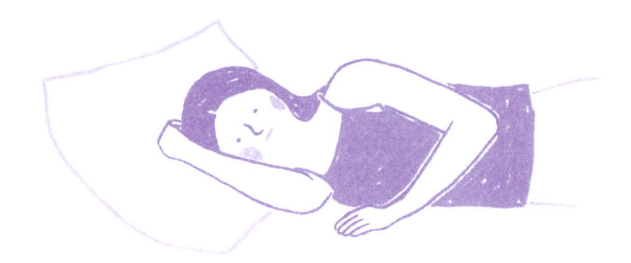

We know that emotions rarely come with reasons, but we still try to define why we fall in love, and find reasons why it has to end when we break up. Maybe it's because we're afraid of being seen as clumsy, immature, or too emotional. Maybe we feel the need to convince our rational mind that our feelings – and the choices that followed – were somehow valid and justified. Maybe we tell ourselves that there must be logic behind it all, so we can prove to others or ourselves that our choices weren't made from feeling, but from reason.

But in the end, those 'reasons' rarely hold much weight – and sometimes, they aren't even true. When emotions fade, so much of what we remember gets re-edited. Looking back, the reasons I once gave for why someone and I 'worked so well' turned out to be nothing more than carefully arranged pieces, stitched together to make sense of something that simply felt good at the time. And then, when I revisit the relationships I should've ended much earlier, I start to notice all the signs that were there that I somehow didn't see back then. The way we interpret the same situation can change entirely, depending on how we feel and what we choose to see. So, maybe we don't need to try so hard to come up with the 'right reasons' just to justify our decisions in a relationship. Reasons are easy to make. Even if you don't have a perfect explanation, all the emotions you feel are always right.

34
Same Moments, Different Memories

Just as history is written by the victors, memories of a relationship are recorded differently by each person.

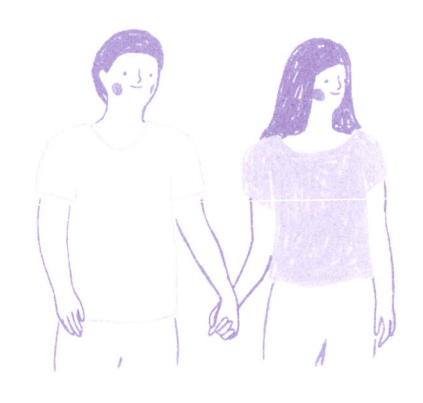

Two people who shared the same moment

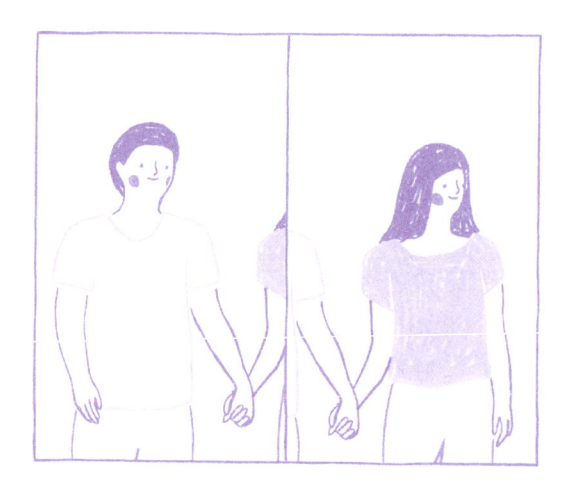

might one day look back from different places at different times,

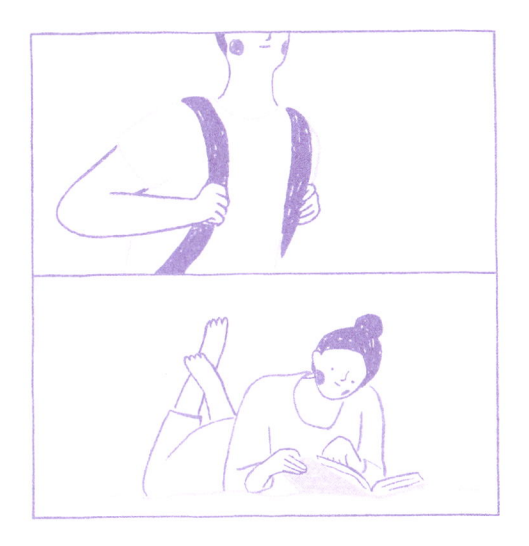

and remember it in entirely different ways.

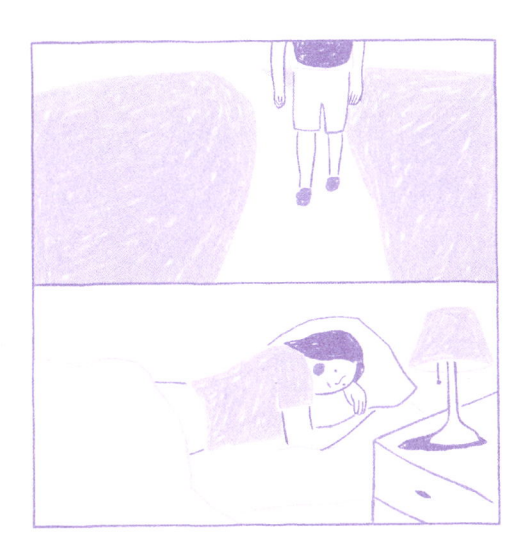

35
Trust the Relationship, Not the Person

The pain of being hurt by someone you trusted

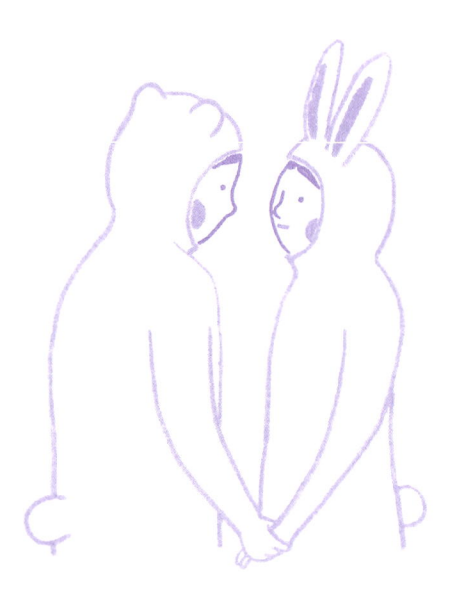

doesn't come only from the hurt itself

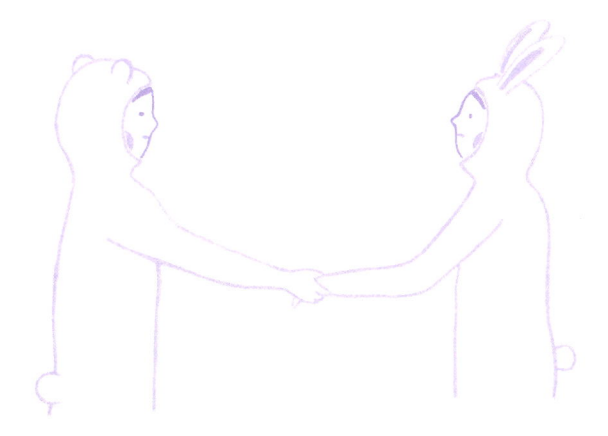

but from the fact that you start to hate the version of you who believed in them in the first place.

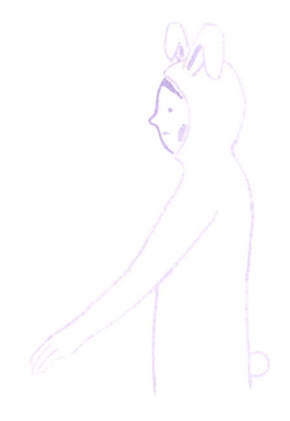

'Trust the relationship, not the person' is one of the rules I live by when it comes to relationships. It's because I believe that no one, myself included, is strong or trustworthy by default. We shift our beliefs or priorities to survive, and no one should be blamed for that.

That's why I choose to put my trust in the relationship, not in the person. I try to fully trust the words and actions that exist within the present connection, while reminding myself that people can always change. This helps me tell the difference between a natural change in someone's behaviour and true betrayal. It keeps me from falling into the trap of labelling myself as a victim whenever someone I trusted lets me down.

Even so, trusting someone wholeheartedly is a rare and beautiful act. If you've ever done that, know that you are already someone deeply kind and worthy.

MY LITTLE TIPS FOR BALANCING HEALTHY BOUNDARIES IN RELATIONSHIPS

If someone you trusted hurt you, don't let the blame fall on you. Let the regret stay with the one who didn't treat your trust with care.

36
Yes, I'm Lonely – But No, I Don't Want to Date

I'm lonely, but I don't want a romance.

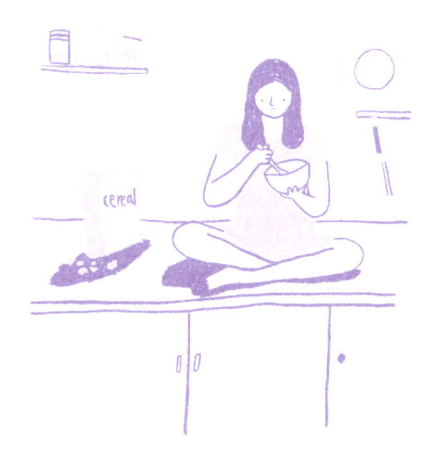

I'm lonely, but I'm not looking for someone to marry.

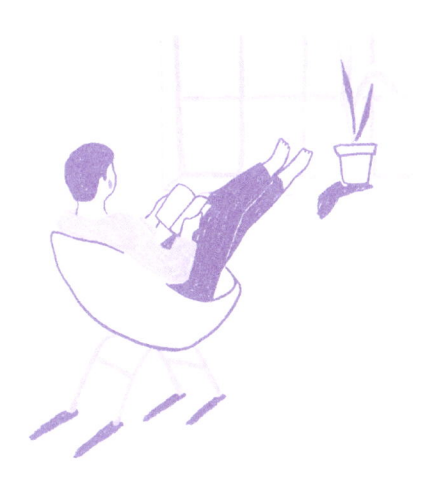

What we

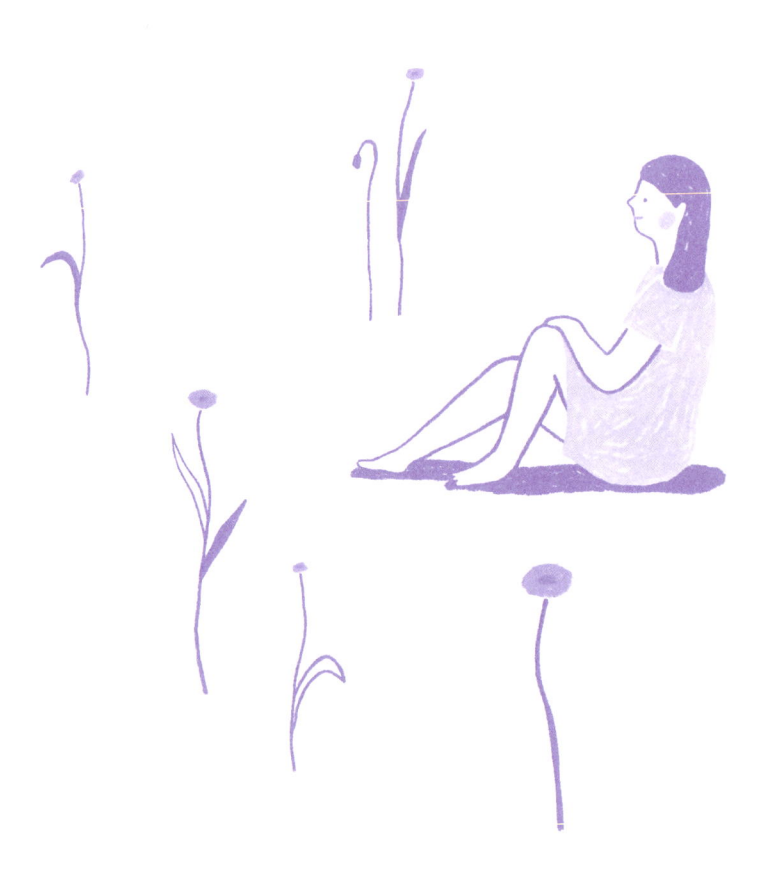

truly need . . .

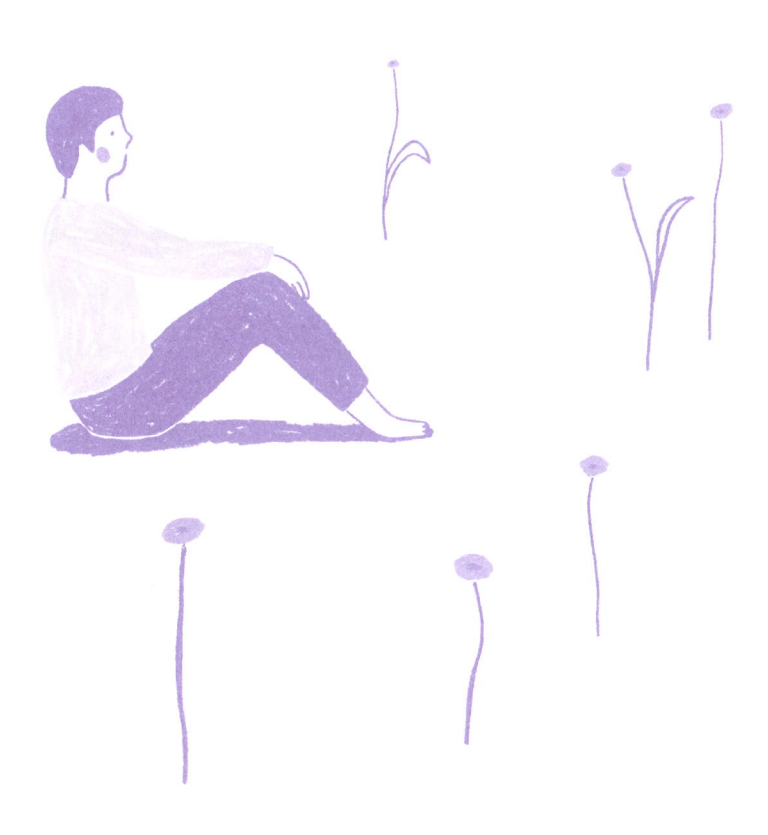

is love.

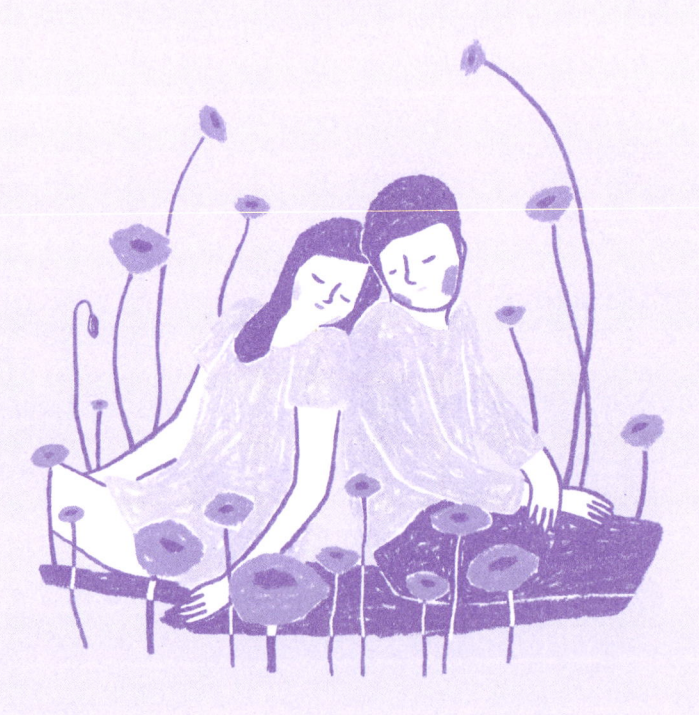

When I see my fine lines deepening or my pores growing larger, anxiety creeps in. The comfort of being alone is often followed by an overwhelming wave of boredom and loneliness, and then I consider trying to meet someone. But when the person across from me seems to want not a life partner but a helper in their life, I find myself closing off again – doubting love, marriage and ultimately, all relationships. I long for the comfort that comes with being with someone, but at the same time, I no longer feel strong enough to carry the many stresses that come with marriage as an institution.

Should I get married? Will life be unbearably lonely and hard if I don't? Can I endure this feeling for decades? Will I ever get used to being alone? Can love or marriage truly fill the emptiness inside me? And why does love always seem to be for dating or marriage?

Maybe I'll never have clear answers to these questions. But there's one thing I've come to understand, based on everything I've experienced so far: the more time I spend in shallow connections, the heavier the loneliness and emptiness become. And that's what frightens me even more – that I'll end up chasing mould for the sake of it, pushed by the pressure to fit into a mould before I've even figured out the kind of love that truly fits me.

Whether it's dating or marriage, I hope love always comes first.

I hope the form we choose to sustain love never becomes the goal itself.

37
I Can Always Choose Better

To bring closure to a past relationship,

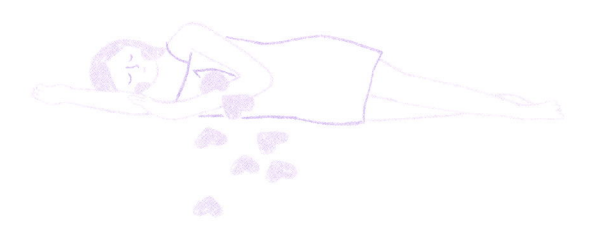

I stopped believing in 'fate' and started believing in 'choice'.

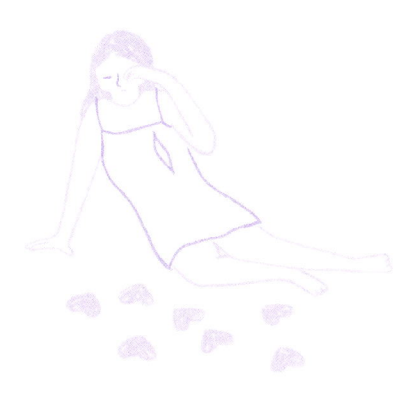

Whether I bury a past relationship as
an unhealed wound,

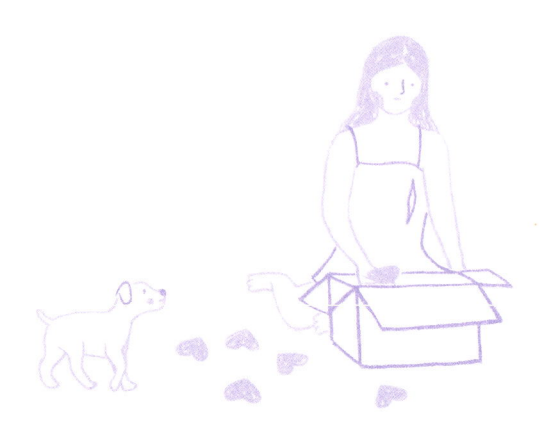

or see it as a series of choices I once made –
that, too, is up to me.

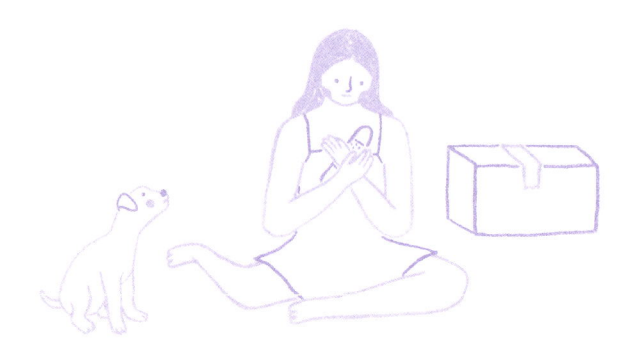

Fate is nothing but the meaning we place on a single coincidence in a sea of many.

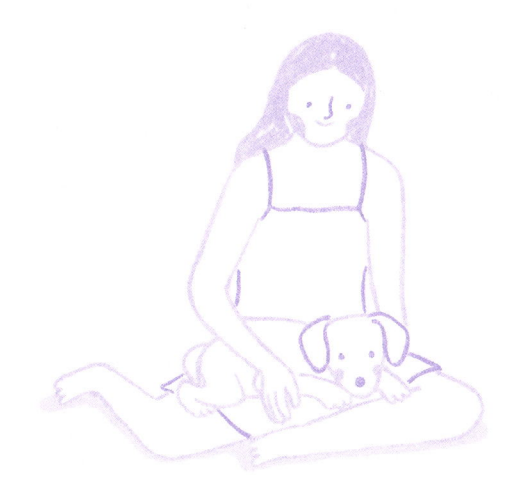

When we look back on painful memories and call them fate, the memory tends to linger as a wound. It's easy to cast ourselves as the tragic protagonist, lost in the sorrow of what once was. But doing so also means telling ourselves that our past self had no power, no agency. That we were merely hurt, helplessly. And from there, it's a short step into victimhood. If we accept pain as something that simply happened to us, we may end up playing a passive role again and again in other relationships, accepting conflict as something we cannot change.

That's why I now choose to believe in choice, not fate, when closing a chapter from the past. To believe in my own choices is to declare that I intend to stay grounded and present in this world and be in charge of my own life. It means I can also choose to open my heart again – not out of fear, but because I decide to.

Who we stay close to, who we let go and how far we keep our distance are all choices we get to make. And even if we make choices we later regret, that's okay, too. Because from every choice we learn, and we can always choose again, and choose better.

38
I Stop Dwelling on Those Who Hurt Me

I've developed a habit of not thinking too deeply about the people who hurt me.

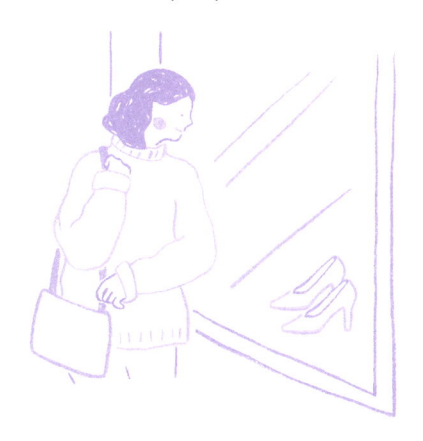

Not because I want to erase the memories – doing so would mean denying who I was.

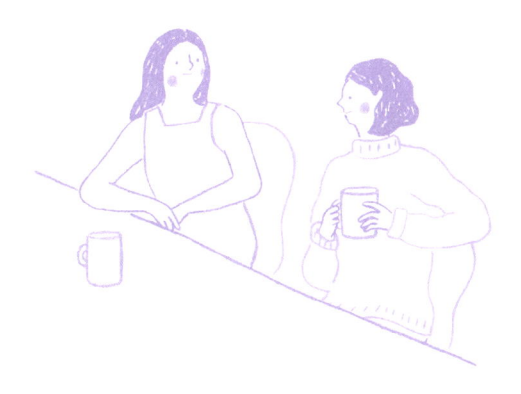

Still, there are some memories
I can only tuck away.

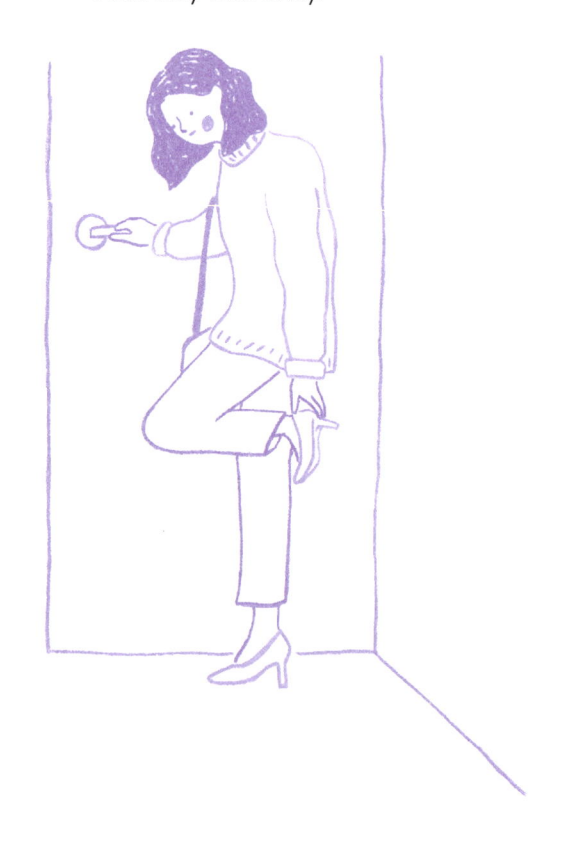

And on the nights when they quietly rise
to the surface,

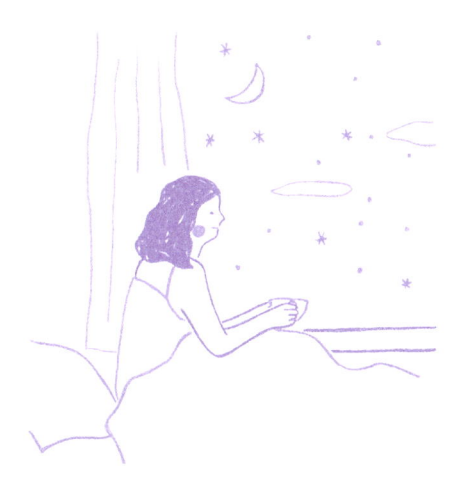

I lie awake, wishing for them to scatter like dust –
softly, without pain.

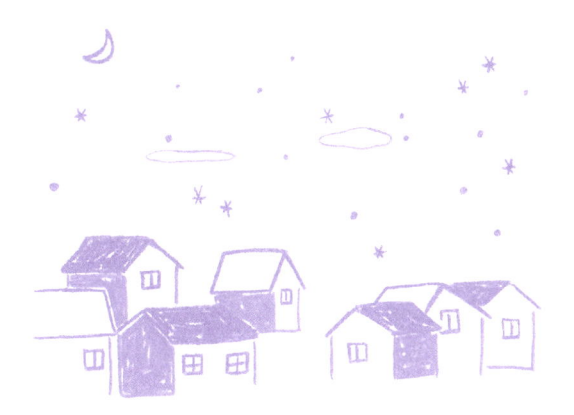

39
The Only One Who Can Embrace Me Unconditionally is Myself

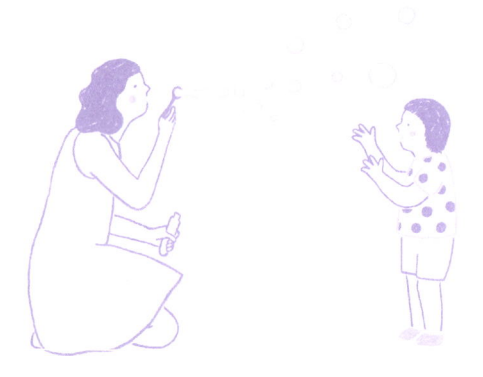

People who didn't grow up with unconditional love

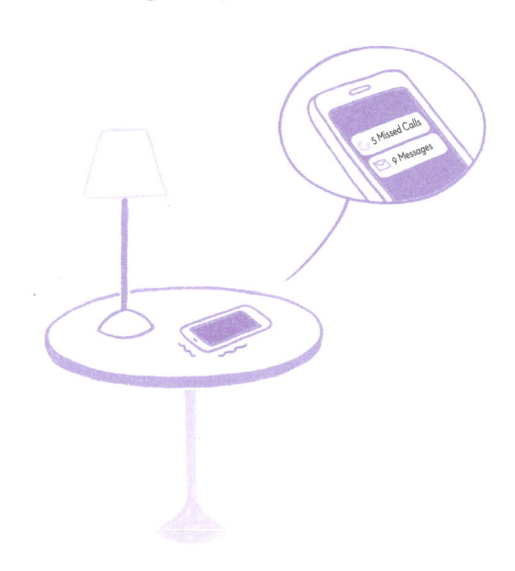

often show specific patterns in intimate relationships.

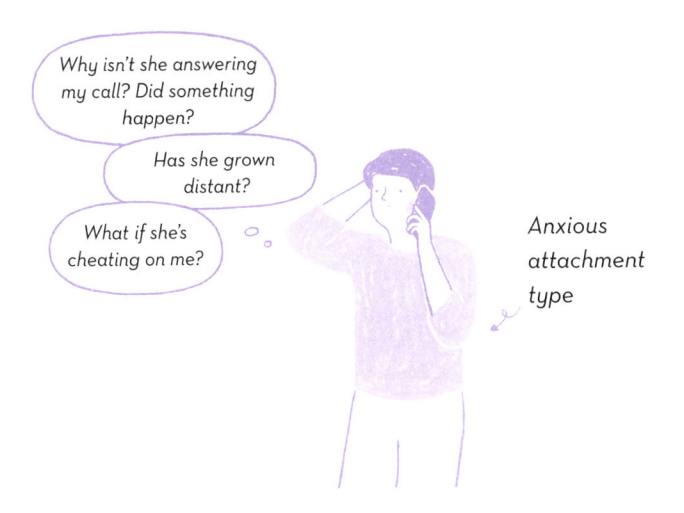

> Why isn't she answering my call? Did something happen?
>
> Has she grown distant?
>
> What if she's cheating on me?

Anxious attachment type

And sometimes, they show behaviours that are hard to understand

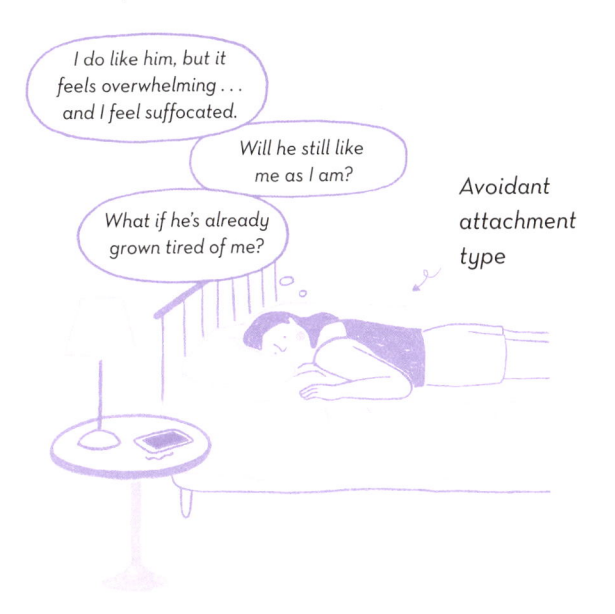

> I do like him, but it feels overwhelming... and I feel suffocated.
>
> Will he still like me as I am?
>
> What if he's already grown tired of me?

Avoidant attachment type

and actions shaped by question marks of insecurity.

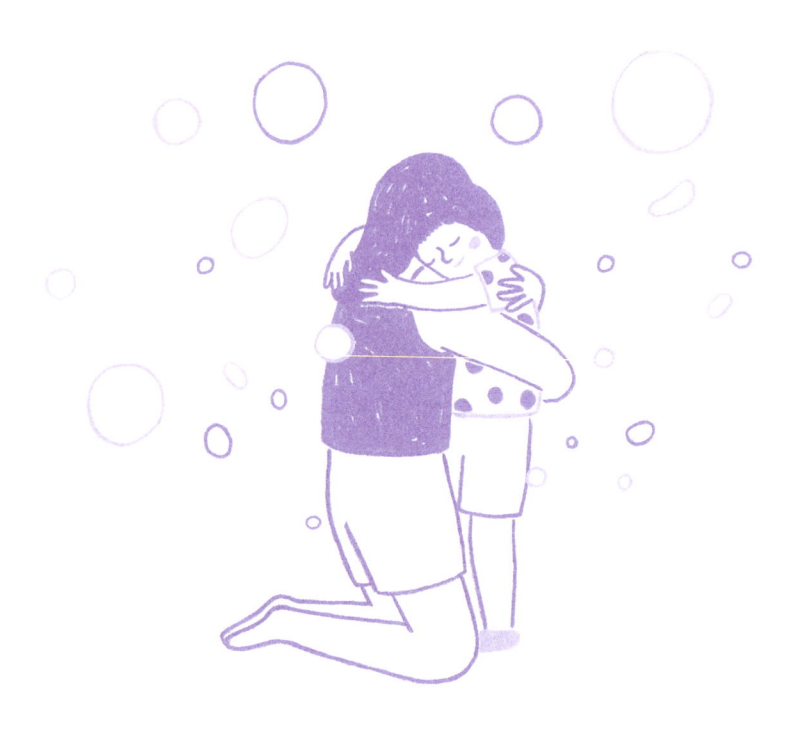

Perhaps the only person capable of embracing me unconditionally is myself.

There are people who, despite managing themselves well in daily life, find their routines falling apart the moment they enter a relationship. They sometimes feel pressured to present an almost perfect version of themselves to their partner, constantly afraid to show any cracks. And some become a completely different person when in a relationship, acting in ways they never would around others – as if testing just how much of their true self their partner can really accept.

The closer the relationship, the deeper the desire for unconditional love and acceptance. Most people share this natural longing. But when that desire crosses the boundaries of what's socially acceptable – or what a partner can reasonably embrace – it can cause cracks to form in the relationship.

Psychologists say these patterns often stem from attachment styles shaped by the quality of unconditional love and acceptance we received from our parents or primary caregivers in childhood. Though well-researched, these theories can sometimes be misinterpreted. If we're not careful, they can trap us in a cycle of blame – unable to move past our parents' shortcomings, remaining stuck in emotional immaturity even as adults.

We cannot change the past. But for the sake of our own growth and healing – and for the sake of building healthier relationships – there comes a time when we must choose to let the past go. You may be an adult now, but the child within you still lingers, waiting. And perhaps the best parent to offer that child the unconditional love they never received is you, and you alone.

40
I Don't Need to Be Liked by Everyone to Be Enough

Rather than striving to be nice to everyone,

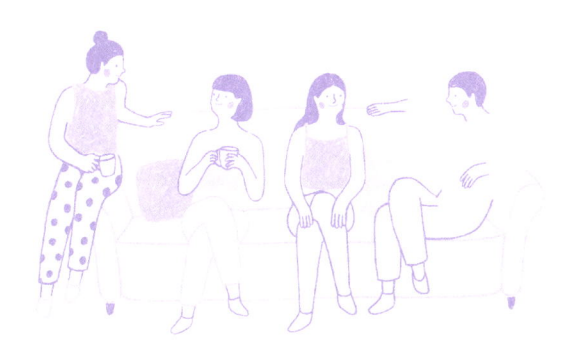

may you learn to recognise how enough you already are – simply by being someone you're proud of.

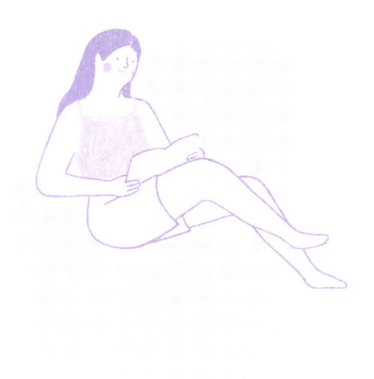

Instead of measuring your worth by the number of connections you have,

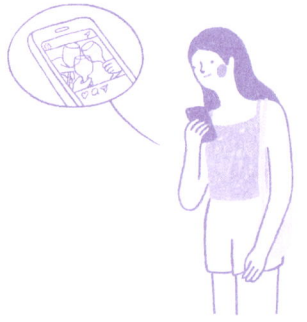

So this is what the cool people's life looks like. Flashy.

may you focus on creating a space where the right relationships can take root.

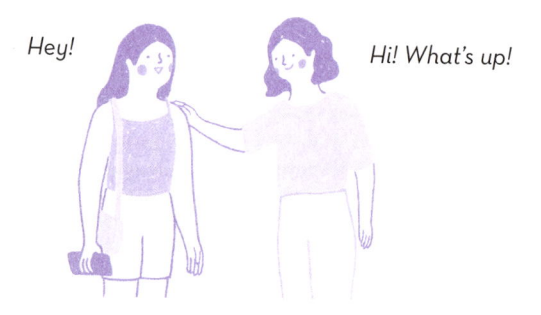

Hey!

Hi! What's up!

May you accept the version of yourself who no longer tries to get along with everyone

That place looks nice! Shall we go there?

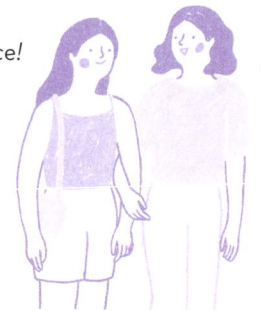

Sure!

and instead chooses to get along with
yourself, above all.

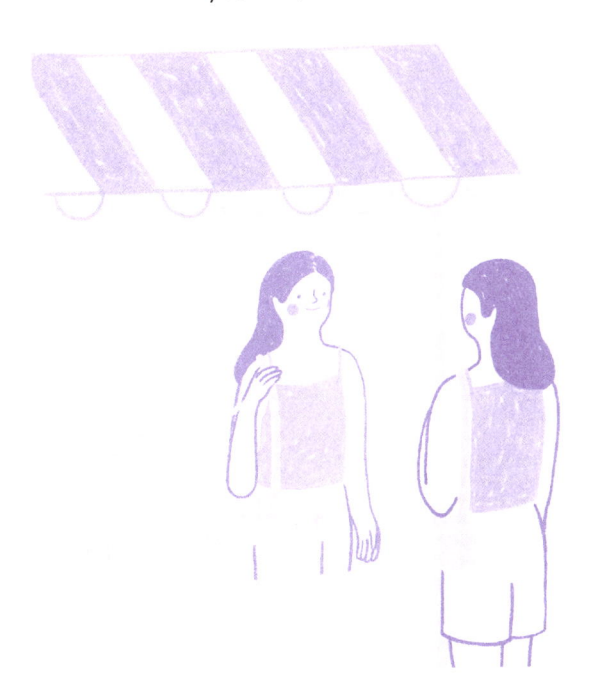

Maybe one of the quiet gifts of growing older is becoming more at peace with things, especially with myself. There are questions I used to instantly blame myself for – small doubts that would have once spiralled into self-criticism. But now, I meet them with a little more compassion. Am I really a good enough person? Did I handle that in a mature, adult way?

Questions like these don't rattle me like they used to. That's because I've chosen to release myself from the burden of needing to be 'the good one' with everybody.

We don't have to be good for everyone. And we don't need to get along with everyone either (aside from the bare minimum required to pay the bills, of course). It's okay to quietly dislike someone and slowly drift away. Whether you're seen as the life of the party or the quiet outsider – it really doesn't matter. What matters is forming relationships that align with who you are and what you value.

Looking back, most of the people I worked hardest to keep around – those I stretched myself thin for – are no longer in my life. If a relationship only survives by being constantly curated, it will eventually dissolve on its own. If I could tell my early twenties self just one thing, it would be that simple truth.

MY LITTLE TIPS FOR BALANCING HEALTHY BOUNDARIES IN RELATIONSHIPS

Chasing relationships just to be seen as a 'good person' in others' eyes is nothing but a waste of precious energy. The sooner you realise that, the wiser – and freer – your life becomes. Before trying to get along with everyone else, never forget: what matters most is getting along with yourself.

41
Singlehood Compensation Bonus

It really feels like all I ever do is give.

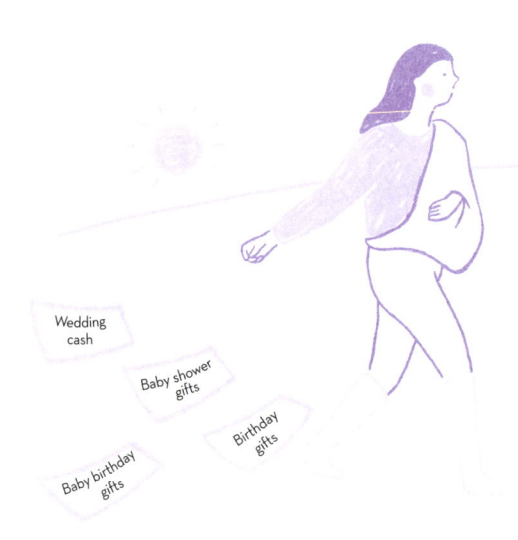

Wedding cash

Baby shower gifts

Birthday gifts

Baby birthday gifts

(A nod to The Sower, a painting by Jean-François Millet).

Everyone gets money and gifts for getting married, for having babies . . .

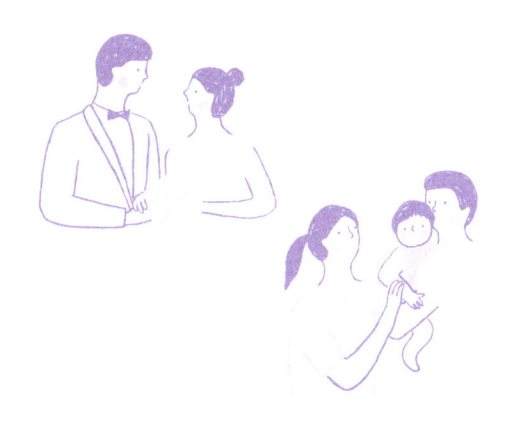

How unfair it is for those of us who are still single!

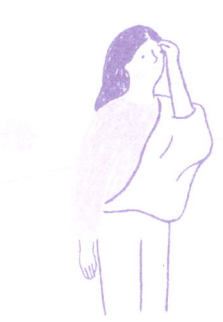

Sigh . . . it's just sweat in my eyes. Definitely sweat. Not tears. Absolutely not.

So let's start a new tradition of celebrating bonuses for singles.

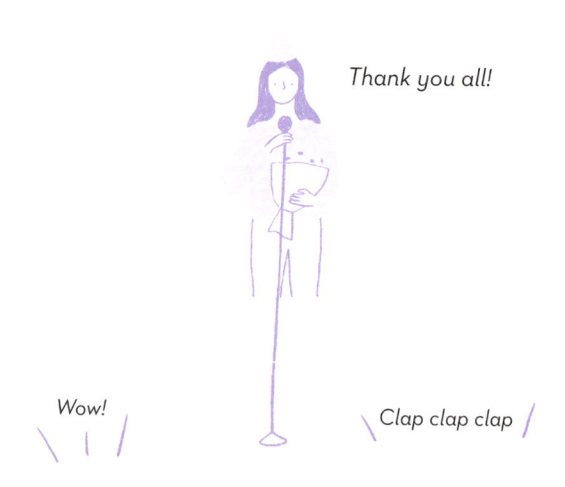

Thank you all!

Wow!

Clap clap clap

Because surviving this harsh world alone deserves recognition.

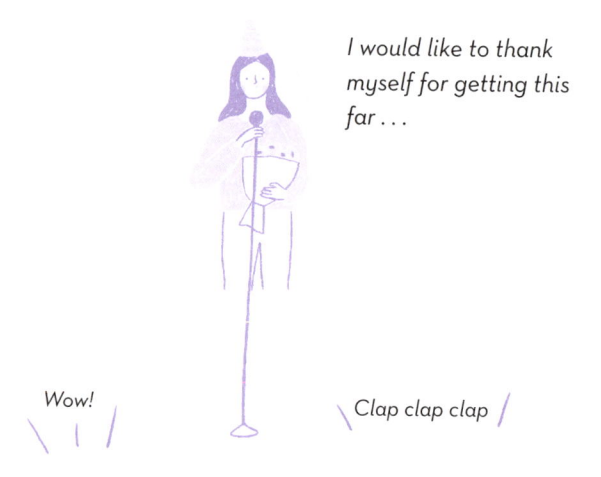

I would like to thank myself for getting this far...

Wow!

Clap clap clap

And a steak, most definitely. That's the most important part.

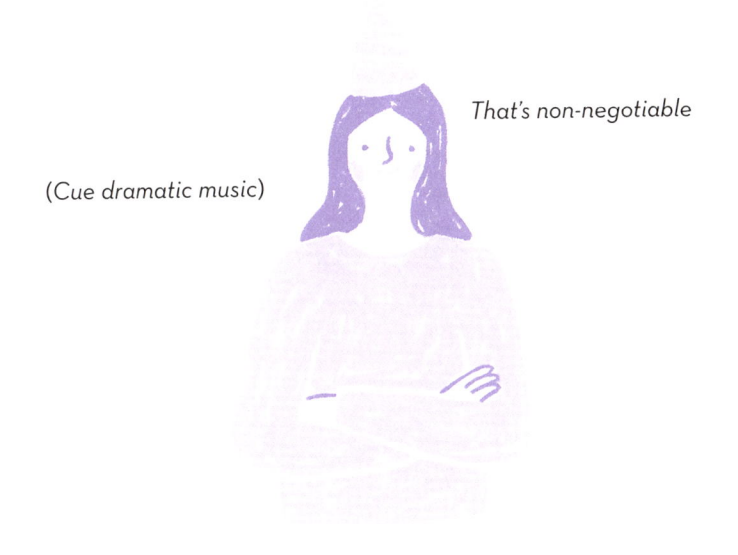

That's non-negotiable

(Cue dramatic music)

42

Certain Things Can't Be Forced – The Human Heart Most of All

At some point, I stopped trying to hold on to people who were ready to leave.

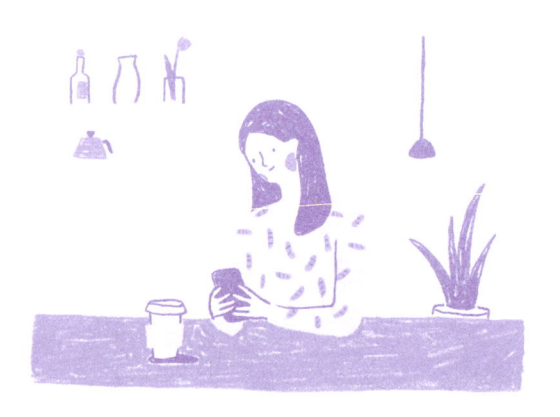

I don't ask for reasons. I don't hold grudges.

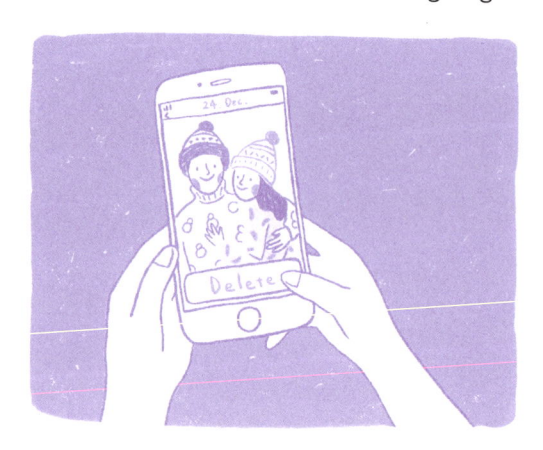

If they're happy, that's enough.

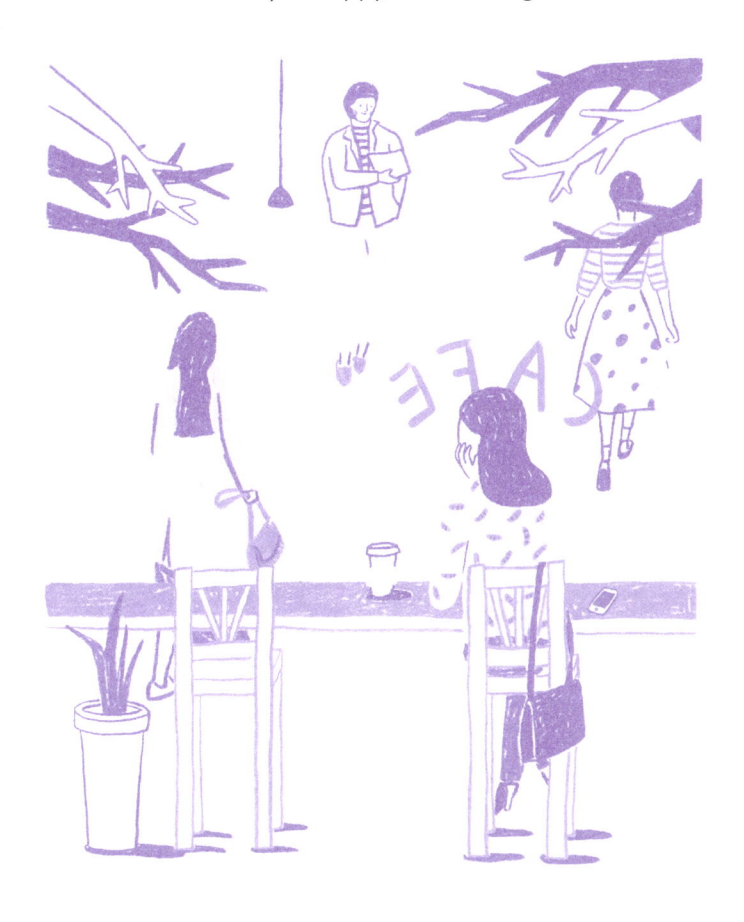

If growing older has taught me anything, it's that the heart is the one thing you can never move by force.

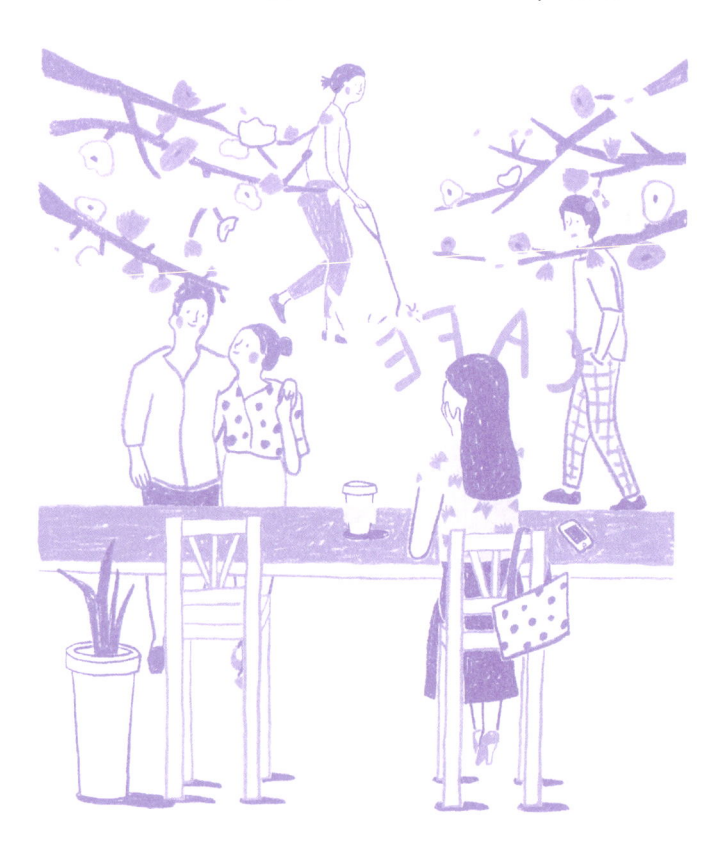

A broken bowl will likely break again. Some connections simply aren't meant to last – maybe they were never truly mine to begin with.

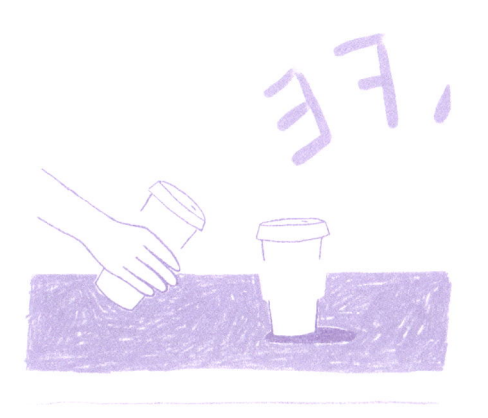

Whether it's true or not, it doesn't matter.

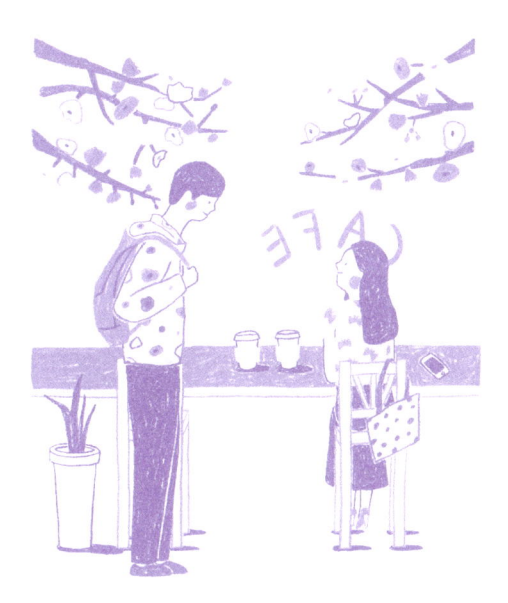

If this perspective works better for my mind,
that's enough for me.

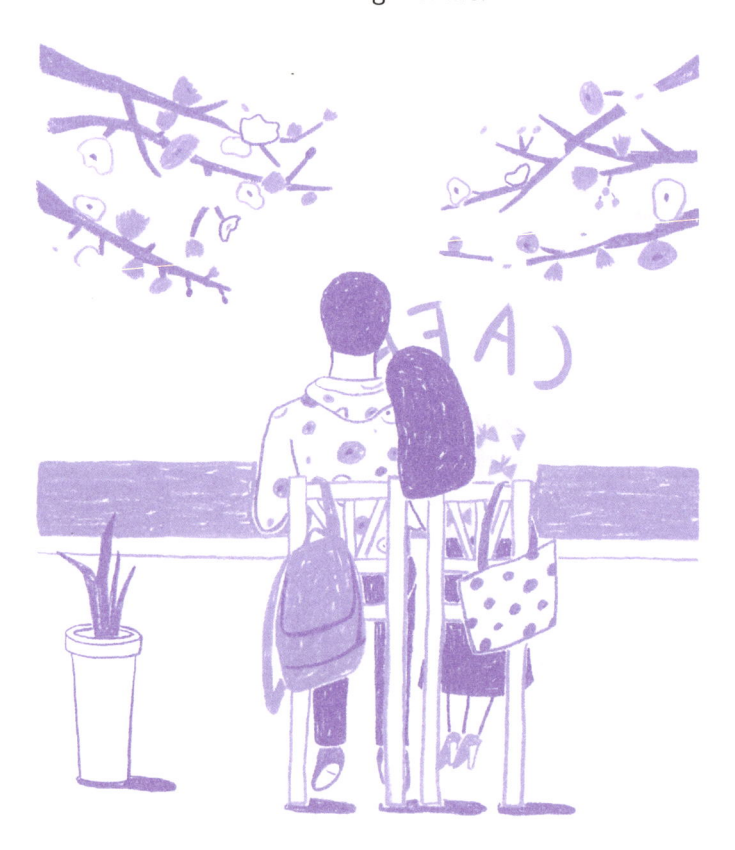

There was a time when I obsessed over questions like, 'Why did we grow apart?' 'Why don't they like me anymore?' Questions without answers – exhausting and ultimately fruitless.

Looking back now, I see there's nothing more foolish than trying to hold on to a heart that's already gone.

Some say you should approach relationships with the mindset of 'Let those who come, come. Let those who go, go.' And yes, if that mindset flows naturally from within, it's probably good for your mental health. But realistically, that kind of detachment? It's a luxury reserved for the enlightened. For people like me – just ordinary, emotional beings – taking that advice the wrong way can lead us down the path of cynicism: 'Forget it. Who needs anyone anyway? Life's a solo act.'

Sometimes our desire to be 'cool' and unfazed in relationships is less about peace and more about escape. A hidden belief that says: If I can't control this relationship, I'd rather be alone than vulnerable.

We spend so much time trying to guess what others are feeling, even when we can't be sure of our own hearts. If I can't even steer my own emotions, how could I possibly grasp – or influence – someone else's?

The heart isn't something you can move with force. It's beyond your control. Instead of pouring energy into someone else's feelings, start with your own. When things don't go the way your heart wants, maybe it's time to follow where the heart can go.

> **MY LITTLE TIPS FOR BALANCING HEALTHY BOUNDARIES IN RELATIONSHIPS**
>
> The heart was never meant to obey. So don't rush ahead of it. Let it move first. May you offer your affection gently to those who come, and learn to let go – more quietly, more calmly – of those who leave.

43
The Heart Locker

When your heart aches too much,

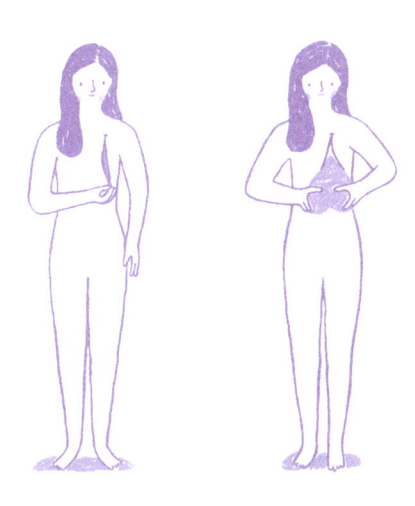

that you wish you didn't have one at all,

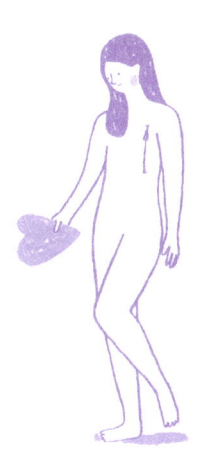

place it for a while in the 'Heart Locker'.

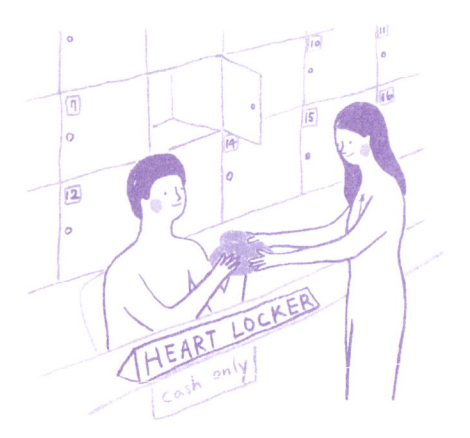

You can come back to reclaim it when you've found the courage to hold the pain again.

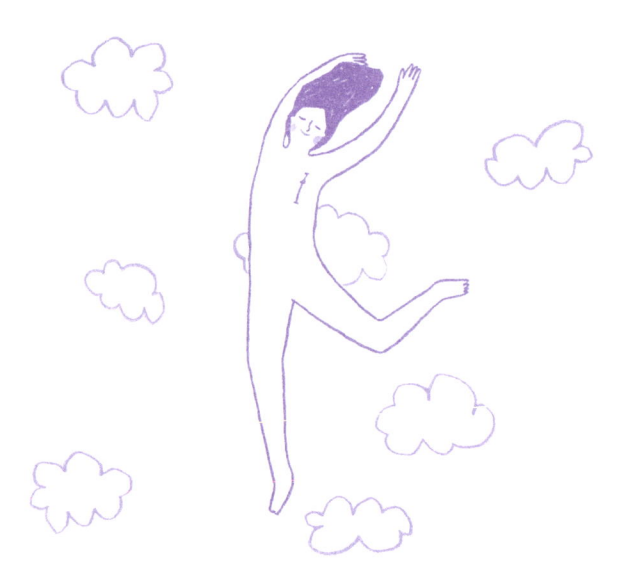

Whenever I'm dealing with work or people who are mentally demanding, I often end up feeling physically unwell. The mind and body are deeply interconnected, and emotional pain often manifests as physical symptoms. In psychology, this is called somatisation – a defence mechanism in which emotional distress takes physical form. It tends to show up more frequently in people who haven't had the chance to process their emotional pain in a healthy way or who have a habit of suppressing it without realising it.

In my case, the signs usually appear as unexplained migraines, digestive issues or bouts of insomnia. On rare occasions, I would have motion sickness I never used to have, ringing in the ears, hives or even toothaches. Oddly enough, when I address the emotional stressor behind it, the physical symptoms often ease on their own. After experiencing this a few times, I've learned to listen to my body when my mind can't quite name the stress yet.

Whenever a new or unfamiliar physical symptom shows up, I immediately stop whatever I'm doing and take a moment to check in with my current situation and relationships around me. (I've realised painfully that this is the most cost-effective way to avoid unnecessary hospital bills.)

Most people experience varying degrees of somatisation at some point in their lives. For example, when your heart hurts emotionally, so deeply that it feels like a real, physical ache in your chest, you might even wish you didn't have a heart at all – or any part of you capable of feeling that kind of pain.

When that happens, it's worth asking: Am I caught up in something too heavy for me to carry right now? Am I keeping someone close who constantly wears down my spirit? What can I realistically do in this moment?

The most important thing is to pause. Step back and take time to reflect. If you can find your own way to let a hurting heart rest, especially in times of conflict or loss, your body will start to feel safe again, too.

44
It's Okay Not to Be Whole on Your Own

Don't you ever get that feeling?

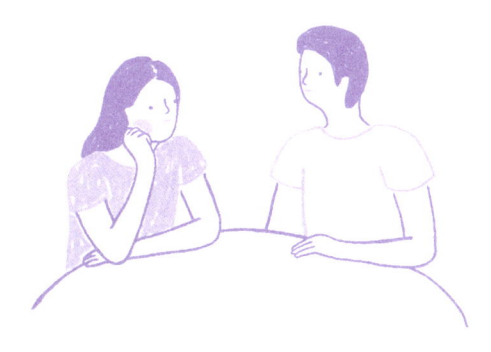

That no matter how many friends we have,
how many people we date,

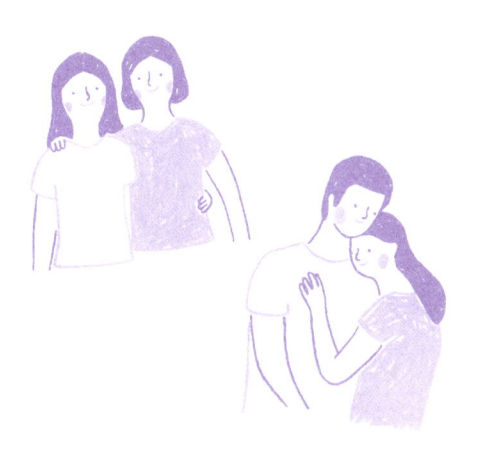

even if we marry or have children,
in the end, we're still alone.

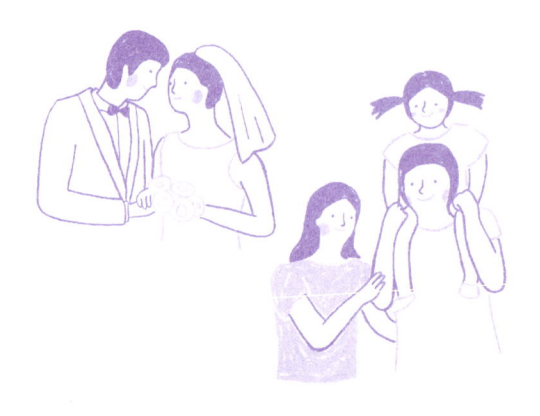

I wonder, can we ever truly get used to being alone?

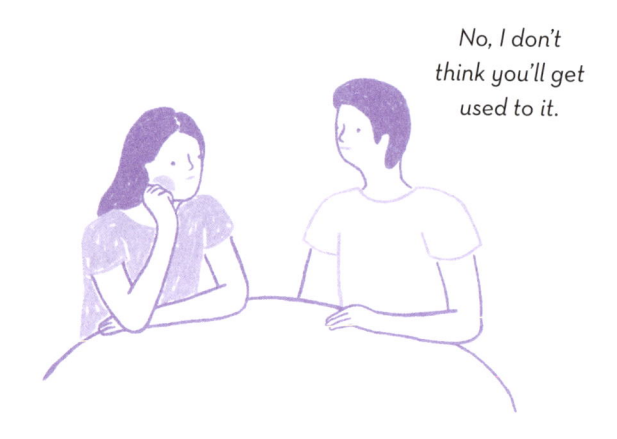

No, I don't think you'll get used to it.

Right now, it's not that you're wondering whether you can get used to it – it's that you simply don't want to.

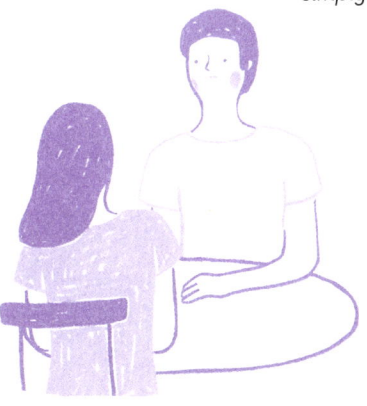

If you don't want to get used to being alone,
you never will.

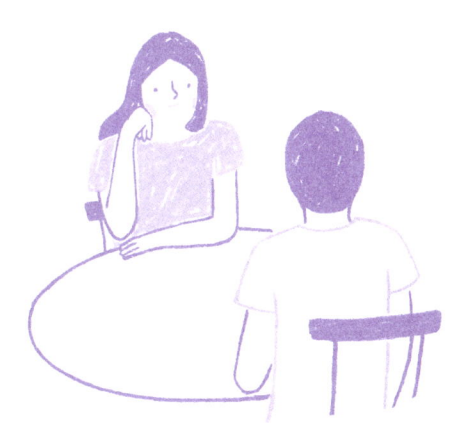

During a solo trip to Jeju in South Korea not long ago, I felt like I was walking around with a Post-it on my forehead that read: Alone. Usually, I've enjoyed the quiet thrill of solitude in a crowd, and I've felt the ache of relative loneliness too – but this was something else entirely.

A kind of absolute aloneness that distraction or comparison couldn't soften.

Yes, there were moments of refreshment, moments that lifted me. But being completely alone wasn't quite as romantic or freeing as I had imagined. Over the course of just a few days, I found myself quickly drained.

They say our brains respond to social disconnection in the same way they respond to physical pain. For humans, wired to survive through connection, getting used to loneliness isn't just a matter of willpower. It's a matter of survival. So if you find it hard to be alone or being alone doesn't feel whole or strong, please don't rush to label yourself as dependent or weak.

Maybe we've misunderstood what it means to be 'alone'. We say we're alone, but how often have we really been alone, completely? And while we sometimes resist solitude with everything we have, we also idealise it, as if true maturity means facing the world on your own.

But in that sense, intentionally placing yourself in a state of deep solitude - a kind of total emotional isolation - can actually be a worthwhile experience. Afterwards, you just might begin to understand how much solitude is right for you and who you truly need by your side.

45
If You Can Be Okay on Your Own

One of those quiet nights on the way home
that feel all too familiar.

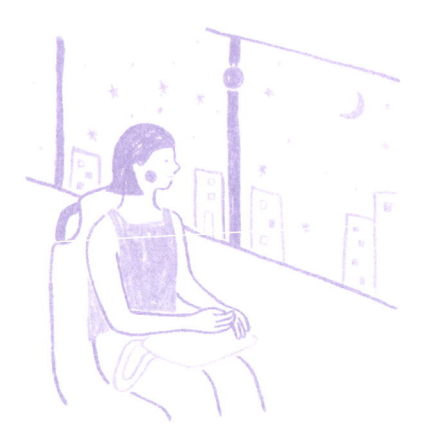

When no one asks if I've eaten or tells me to get home
safe. No one nags me about anything.

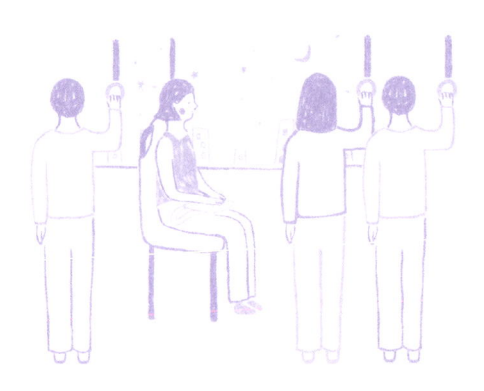

The only thought that passes through my mind is how beautiful the neon lights are.

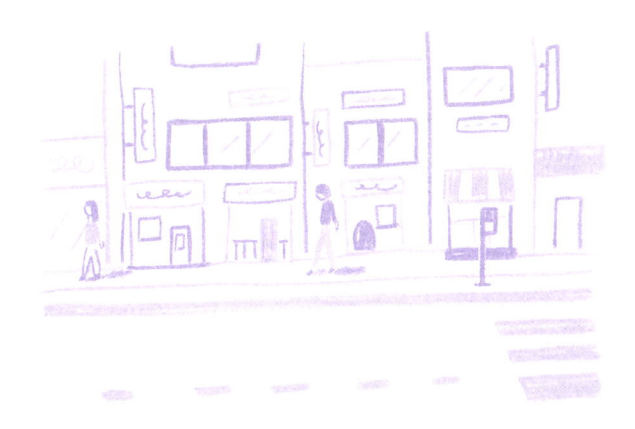

They say if you can be at peace on your own, you'll be able to be at peace with others, too.

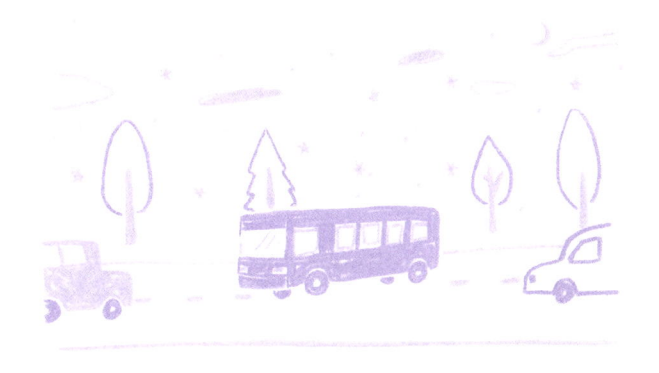

Maybe now . . . I'm finally ready to be at peace with someone.

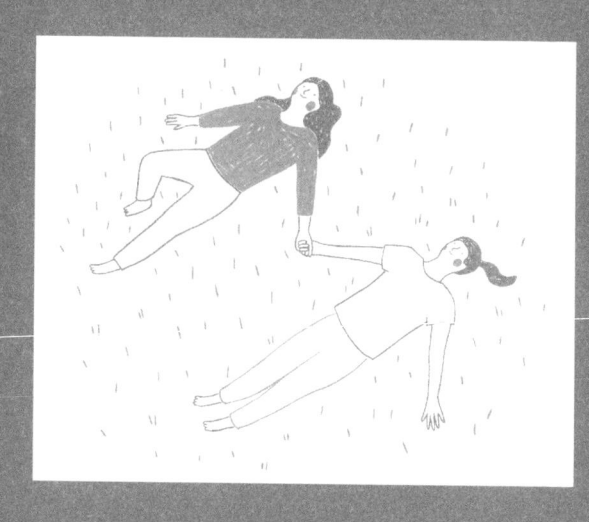

PART 03

PEOPLE ALWAYS
NEED PEOPLE

46
There's an Invisible Line Between You and Me

I'm being kind to you,

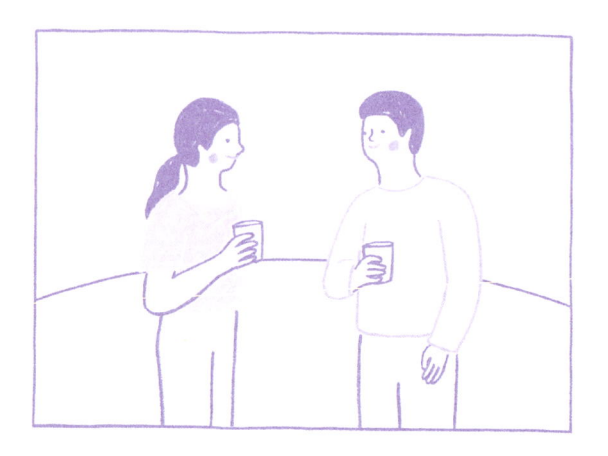

but that doesn't mean I want to get closer.

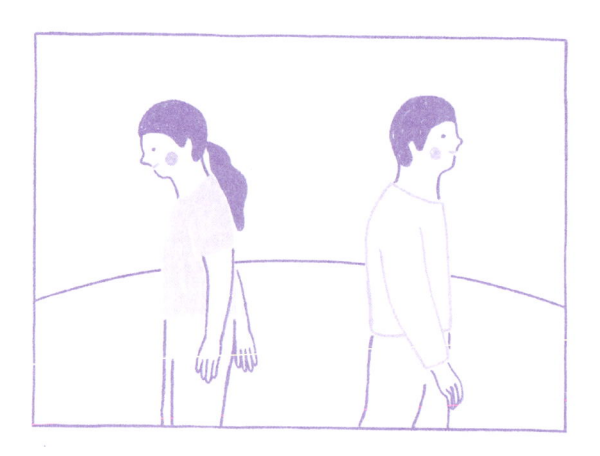

I want you to like me more,

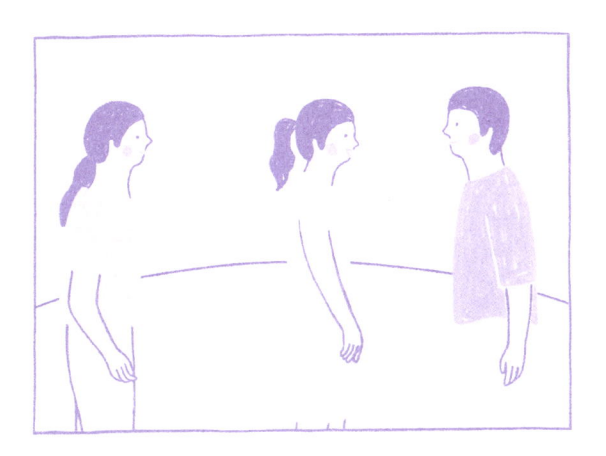

but I don't want to like you back. Does that make me selfish?

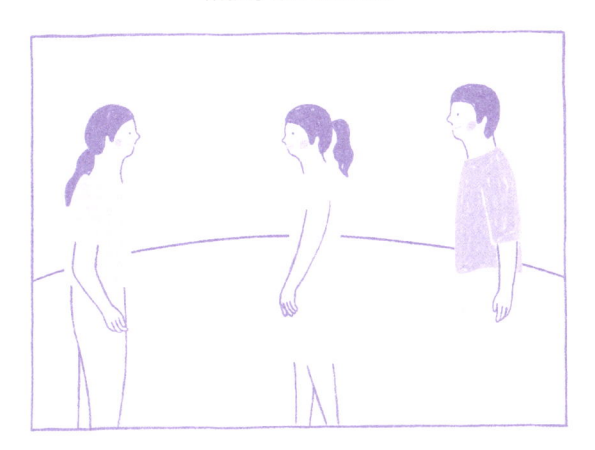

I'm afraid that the more time we spend together, the more I let myself care about you,

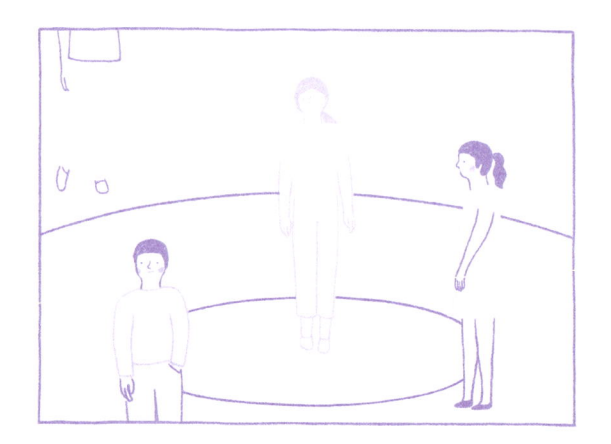

the more I'll start to lose who I am.

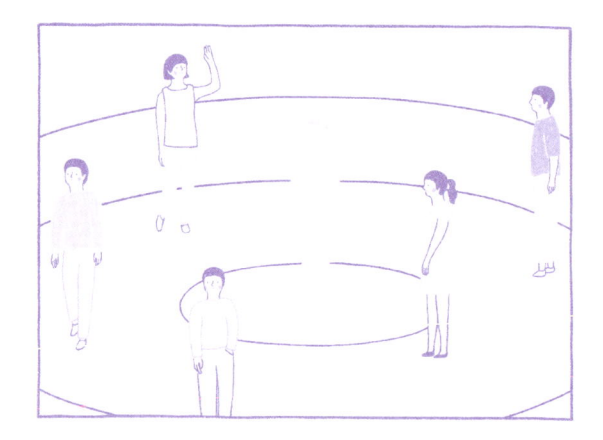

I often set invisible boundaries with my friends and acquaintances, depending on how emotionally close I feel to them. Of course, I don't write them down in a journal or say them out loud. But when someone asks me for help, or when I have to choose whose plans to prioritise, those lines I've drawn always come to mind.

Psychologists say that maintaining a healthy emotional distance in relationships helps protect your sense of self and supports overall wellbeing. In that sense, maybe I'm doing it right.

But when someone stands just outside the circle I've drawn around myself, inviting them in can feel impossibly difficult. Even with those I consider close, I find myself thinking about where the boundary is, sometimes even obsessing over it.

Whenever someone even inches past that invisible line, my guard goes up, afraid I won't be able to protect myself. And so, even with those I'm closest to, it feels as if there's an invisible wall between us.

What exactly am I so afraid of? And when will I have the courage to let someone cross that line and draw near?

47
The Art of Being Not Too Close

Sometimes, it's the relationships that aren't too close

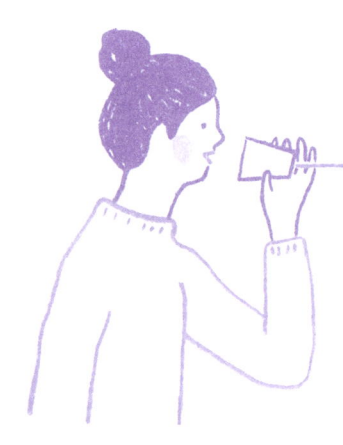

that last the longest.

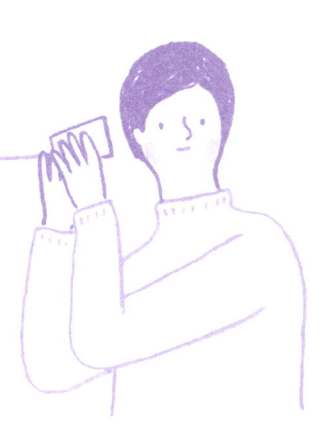

Because intimacy always comes with

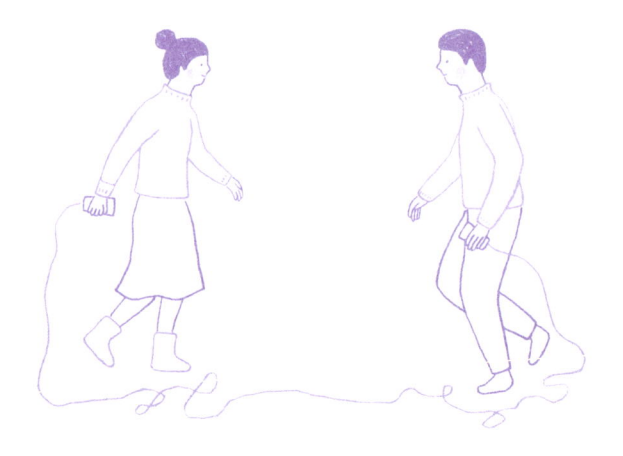

expectations and, therefore, disappointment.

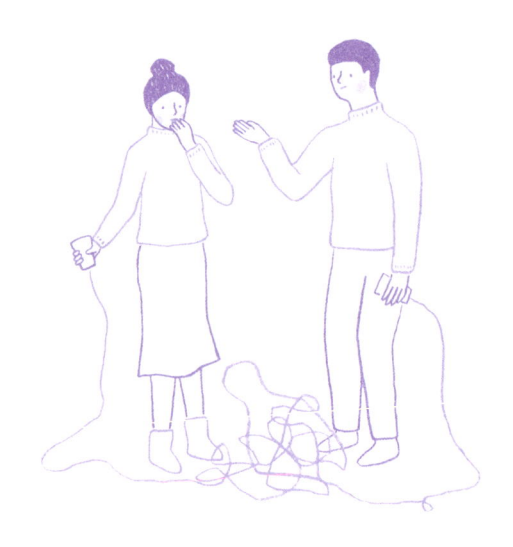

The more we grow close, the more tangled things can become.

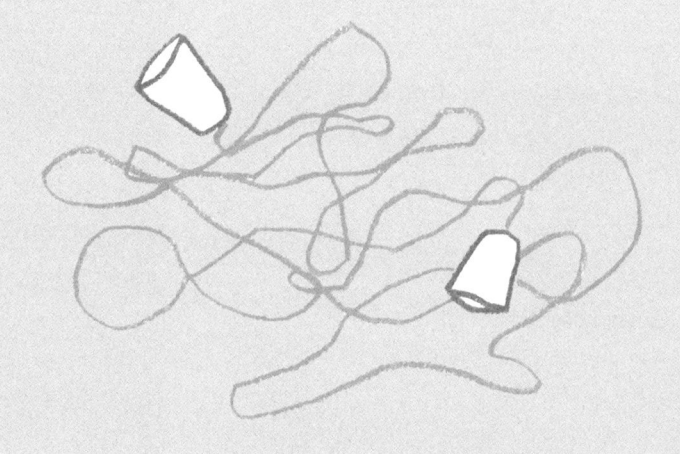

Work colleagues, friends with shared hobbies, acquaintances I know through others – these connections accumulate over time. And while I want to be a responsible adult who stays genuinely engaged in all of them, it's not easy for someone like me, who naturally leans towards the quieter side of social life. I am torn between wanting to prioritise the people I truly care about, and not wanting to disappoint – or lose – anyone at all.

But relationships aren't something you can build alone. No matter how much effort I put in, I can't control what the other person wants when it comes to closeness, and I certainly can't go deep with everyone. That's why, sometimes, a quiet kind of skill is required: the ability to maintain a connection that's neither too close nor too far. Because if the thread between us is pulled too tight, it might snap. And if it's too loose, it might tangle beyond repair.

MY LITTLE TIPS FOR BALANCING HEALTHY BOUNDARIES IN RELATIONSHIPS

Not too much, not too little. Not too close, not too distant. Not too cold, not too warm. Depending on the moment, let's become relationship nomads – drifting gently into whatever kind of closeness feels right at the time.

48
The Right-sized Gap in the Heart

When the thread that once tied you and me together breaks,

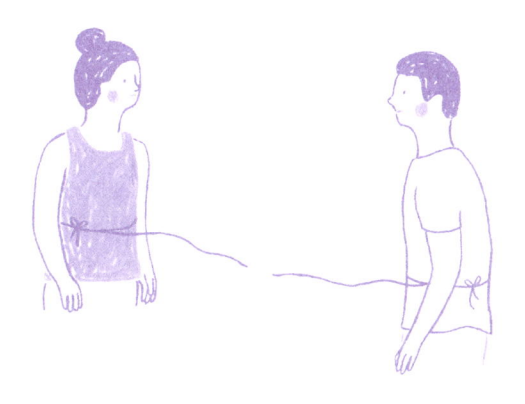

I gather those frayed strands and start weaving them into a shield to protect myself.

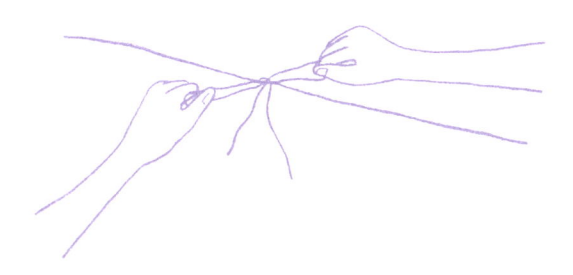

Once that shield grows thick and strong, I no longer get hurt by every fleeting connection.

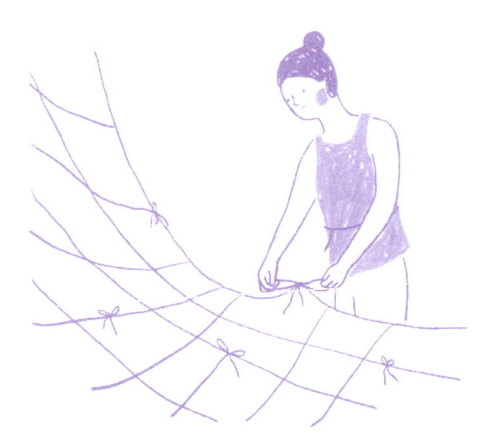

But at the same time, I struggle to let anyone in.

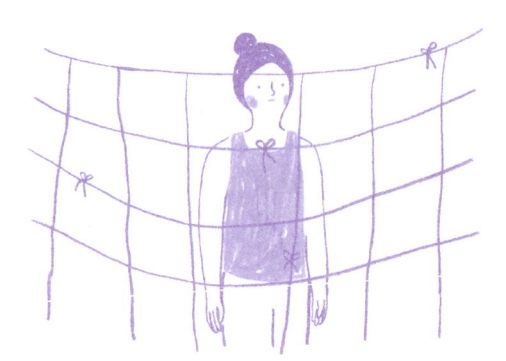

That's when good friends become the ones who gently make space – little openings in that shield.

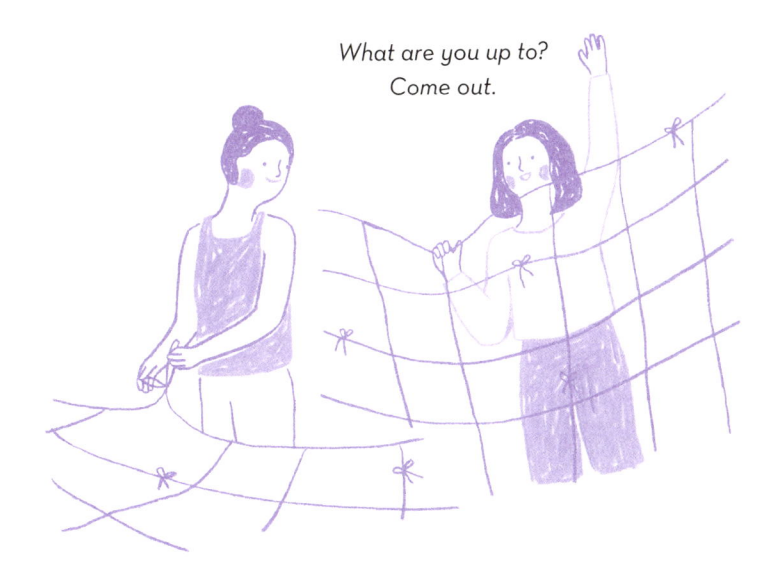

What are you up to? Come out.

49
Somewhere Between Alone and Together

When no one texts me, I feel lonely.
But when they do, I feel bothered.

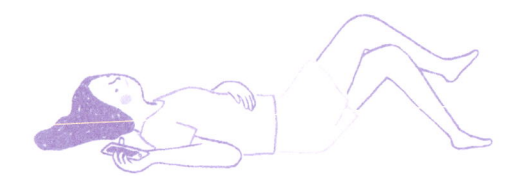

Being with others drains me quickly, but being alone makes me feel empty.

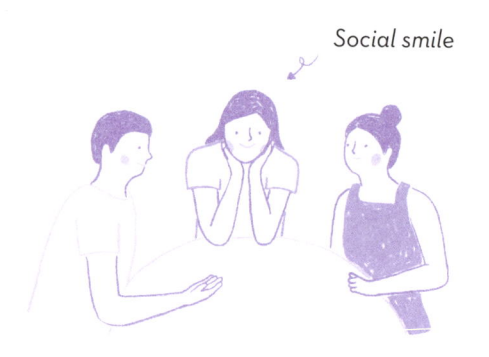

Social smile

There are more and more days like this lately -

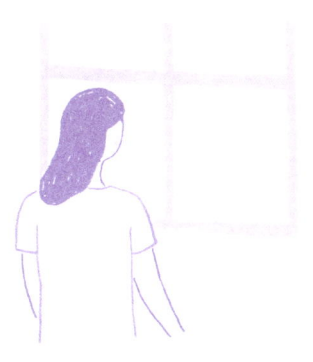

days when I'm not fully whole on my own, yet somehow
still unable to be fully with someone else.

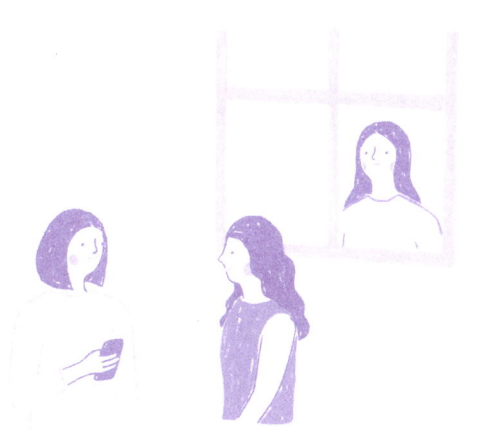

Some people have a low sensory threshold. They feel cold easily, but just as quickly, they overheat. Their bodies respond rapidly to changes in their environment.

And then there are those with a low emotional threshold. When surrounded by people, they become easily overwhelmed. But when left alone, loneliness sets in just as fast. Their feelings swing from one extreme to the other, and they reach the limits of their emotional capacity in a flash. They know they're not quite whole on their own, but being immersed in connection can feel equally exhausting.

Still, even the most emotionally sensitive among us need intimacy. They just might need to approach it differently, like parallel play, a term from early childhood development describing when children play side by side, together, yet separate.

People like this thrive in a relationship that respects space. Time spent side by side, without pressure or intrusion – a quiet kind of togetherness. Maybe this way, I can stay close to the people I care about, without giving up the time and space I need for myself.

50
No One is Truly Indispensable

Everyone has a limit to how many relationships they can hold.

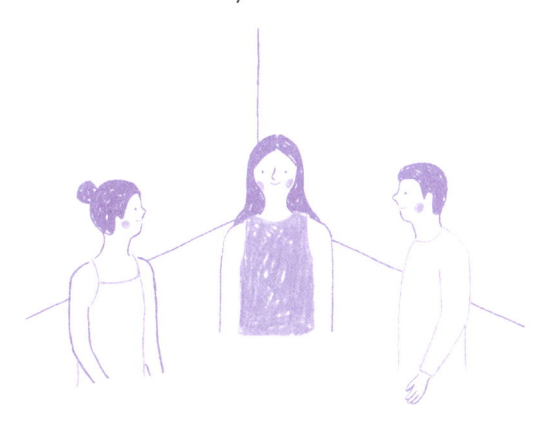

And when that space is full, you have to let someone go before you can let anyone else in.

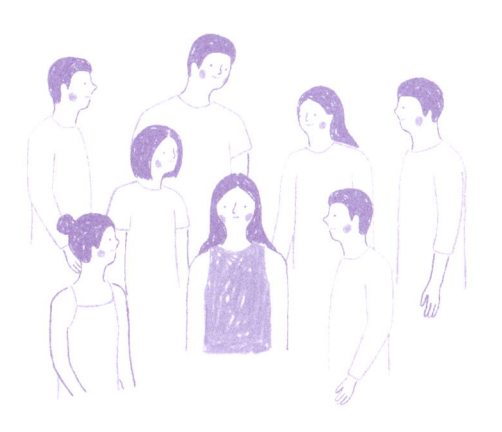

There is no one in this world you absolutely can't live without.

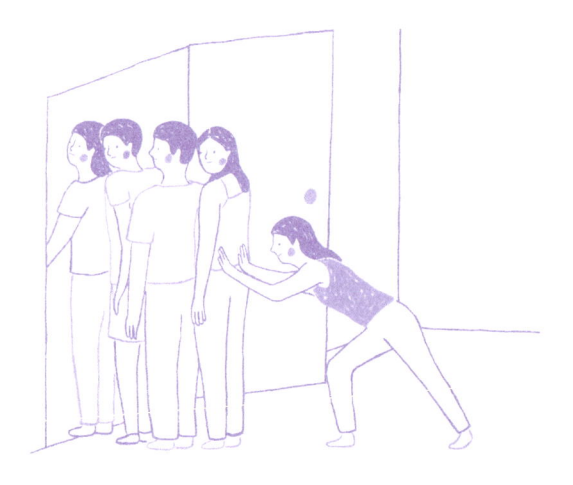

You have to be able to walk away from those who don't respect you.

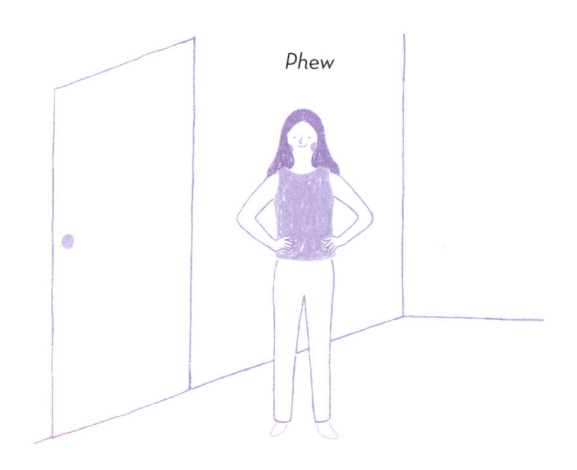

Phew

That's how you make room for someone
who does to come in.

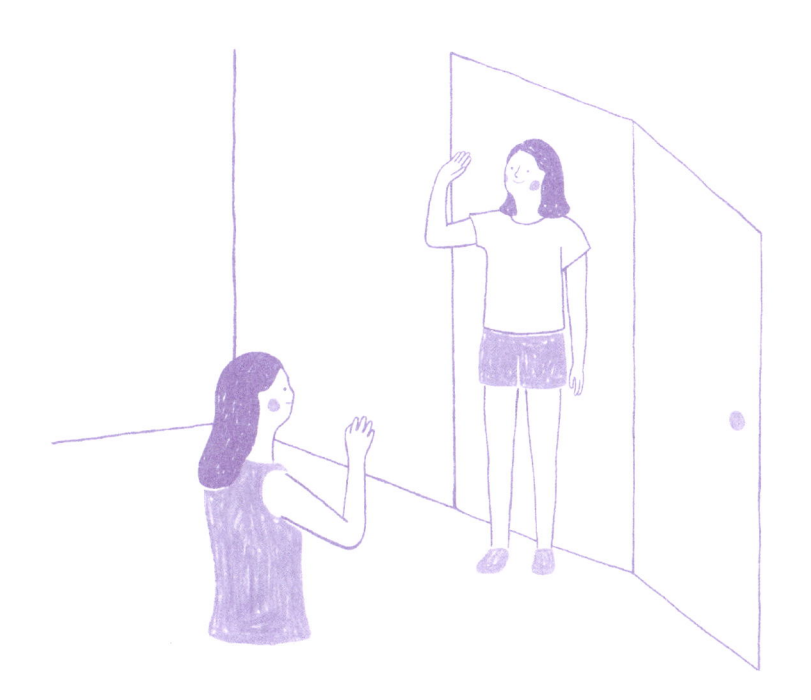

When my self-esteem was low, I realised that I was surrounding myself with people who disrespected me. At the time, I accepted it as normal. And honestly, that was the better version of me. When my self-worth hit rock bottom, I took it even further – blaming myself entirely for the way others treated me.

I thought it was because I was selfish. After all, I didn't know how to sacrifice enough for others. (Some people even gaslighted me into believing that, especially those who wanted me to keep sacrificing.)

But even if it leaves an empty space at first, it's better to let go of anyone who makes you feel small or unworthy. Just because you're hungry doesn't mean you should fill yourself with food that doesn't nourish you.

People who disregard your needs or speak carelessly should be filtered out early, before you get used to calling that kind of relationship normal. Any connection that requires your constant self-sacrifice isn't equal – and it's not meaningful, either.

MY LITTLE TIPS FOR BALANCING HEALTHY BOUNDARIES IN RELATIONSHIPS

When you clear out the space taken up by relationships that don't respect you, the emptiness that follows can become the very opening through which better people find their way in.

51
When Someone Enters Your Heart

When you let someone into your heart,

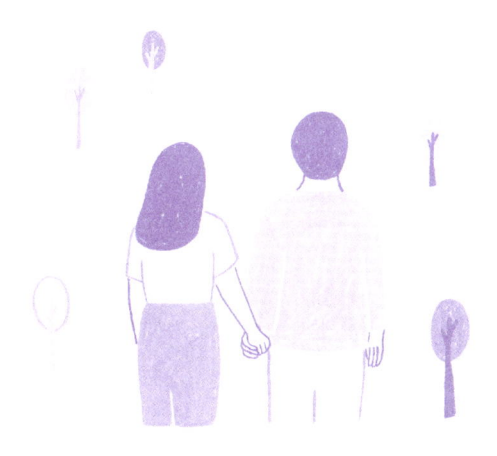

everything begins to remind you of that person.

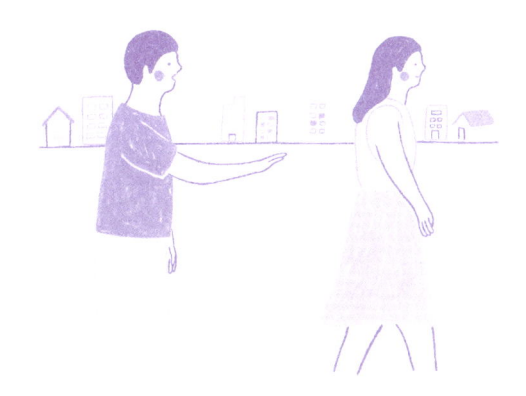

You catch glimpses of them in strangers passing by.

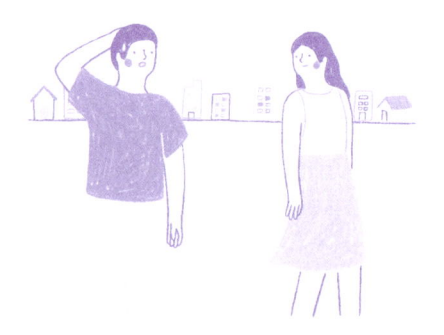

In a celebrity whose smile feels just like theirs.

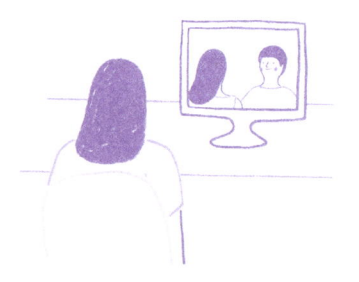

In a scent that lingers just like they do.

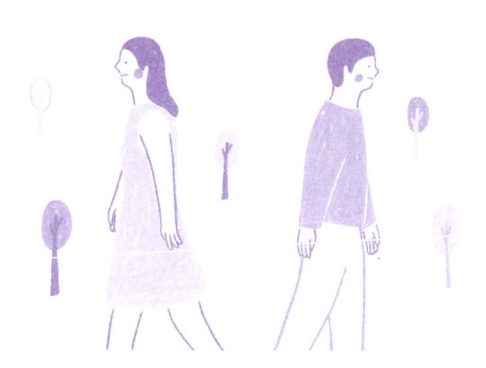

52
When Excitement Alone Doesn't Feel Like Enough

Should I keep seeing him?

Why not? It's not like he's asking you to marry him now.

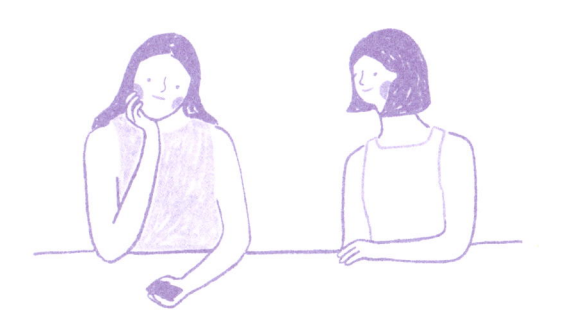

I feel like he expects too much from me, and I'm not sure I'm good enough.

Hey, you are a good person. But if he constantly needs reassurance, that does sound exhausting.

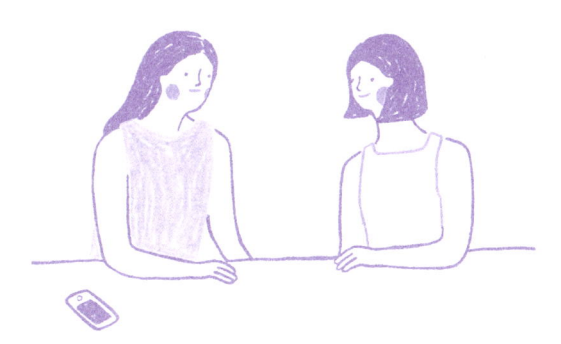

I do like him. But I'm worried that if I open my heart, I don't know if I'll be able to handle what comes next.

Maybe... your feelings just aren't big enough to outweigh the anxiety.

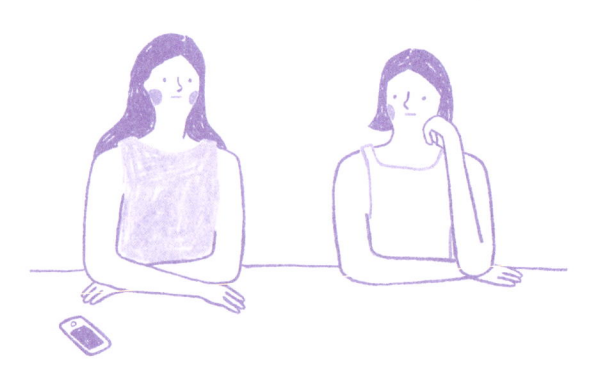

And maybe you simply learned that liking someone isn't always enough.

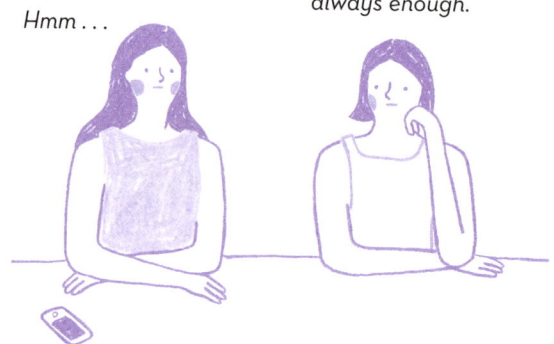

Hmm...

It's getting harder to open my heart to someone new. I don't want to blame it on age, but maybe it is that, at least in part. Not the number itself, but the fact that I've watched the same story play out too many times. Now, when someone says just a few lines, I predict the ending before the story begins. Call it experience, if you will – but sometimes, it just feels like premature cynicism.

Even when I start to like someone, I can't enjoy the excitement. The worry comes first. Then the fear. I've learned the hard way that feelings don't know how to stop halfway. Once they begin to grow, they grow beyond control. And maybe that's why – because I'm not sure I can manage what I'll feel, I hesitate to trust.

When the thrill of meeting someone new isn't enough to give you courage, maybe it helps you step off the stage of life and become a quiet observer.

Take one step back. Watch the story unfold. See what happens next. It might be a more interesting story than you imagined.

53
When We're Meant to Cross Paths

We often find ourselves most alone when
we don't want to be.

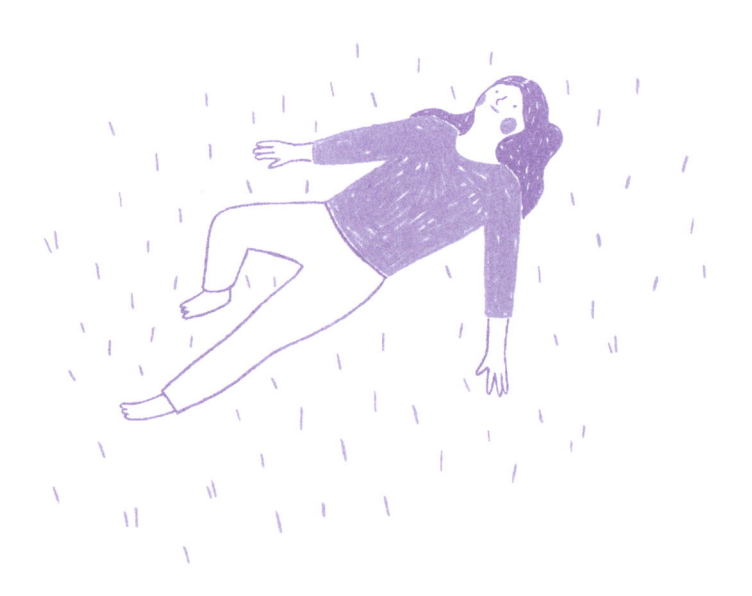

Sometimes, when we want to be alone,
someone reaches out for help.

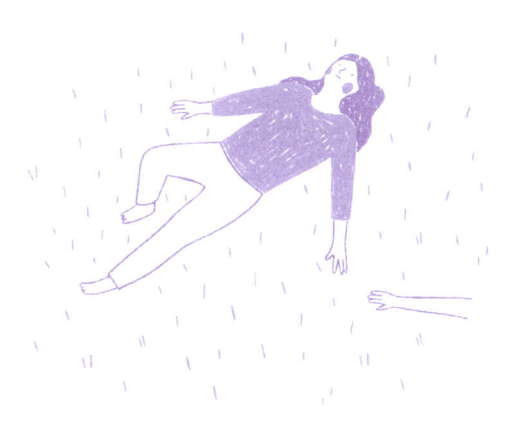

And ironically, it's often the moment we choose solitude
that we realise that we're not alone.

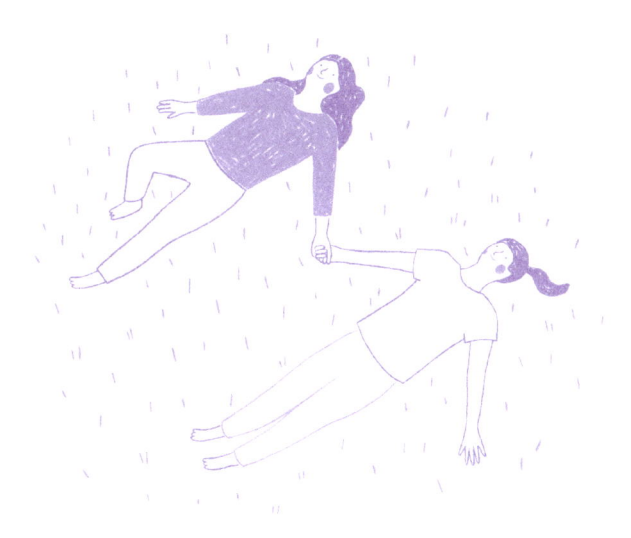

54
Maybe, Just Once, It's Okay to Give My Whole Heart

We gotta date a lot when we're young!

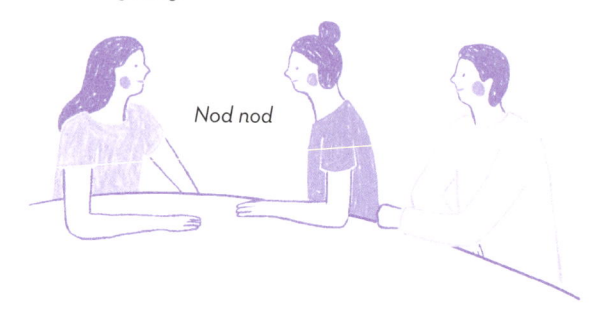

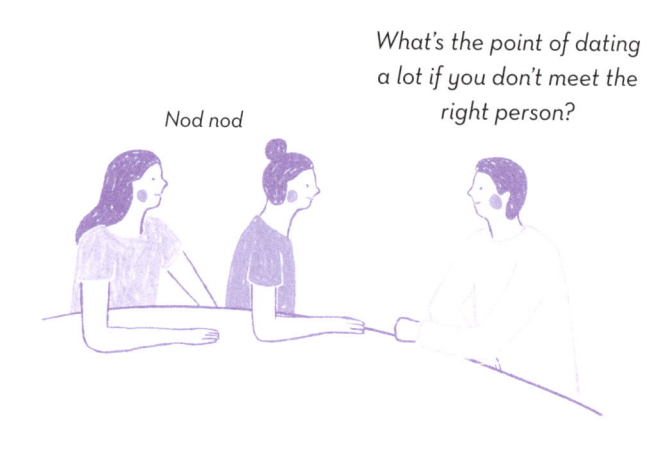

Nod nod

Nod nod

What's the point of dating a lot if you don't meet the right person?

*I think what matters most is letting
yourself fall in love completely –
at least once in your life.*

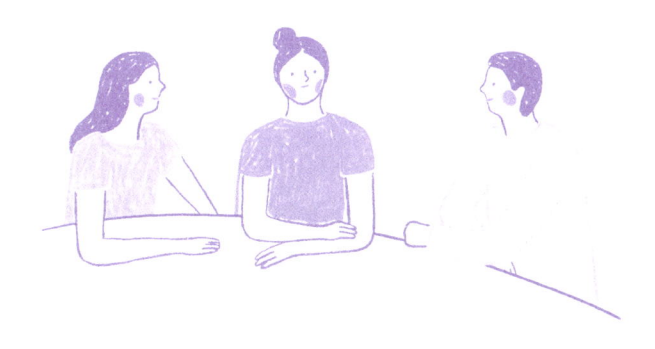

*It's the only way to really
understand how much of yourself
you're willing to share again.*

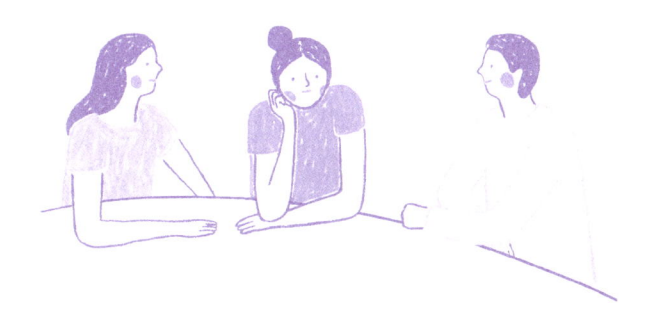

The only truly good thing a finished relationship leaves behind is this: you grow – if only by the weight of what you've been through. Because I've learned how to carry my emotions more carefully, I don't throw my whole heart in so recklessly anymore. Now, my body knows my whole being senses the moment when it's time to hold back, to stop my restless heart from rushing in too far.

No matter who I meet, the one constant in every relationship is me. Through each relationship, I came to know a slightly different version of myself. There's always something to learn, always a way to grow. It's a bit like drinking – you have to experience brutal hangovers once or twice to really learn when that one last drink becomes too much.

So if you haven't yet given your heart completely, maybe it's okay to try, at least once.

Because no matter how things end, every relationship leaves behind a lesson to learn.

55
Choosing to Let Go of the Time We Shared

At some point in my life, I stopped keeping up with
the daily lives of old friends.

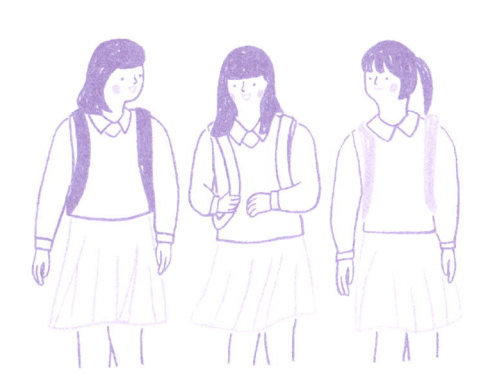

Is this just part of getting older?

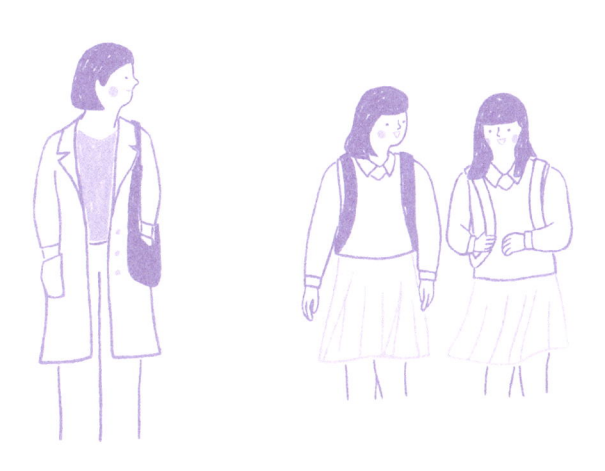

As we've grown apart, the fewer shared interests, the fewer reasons to reach out.

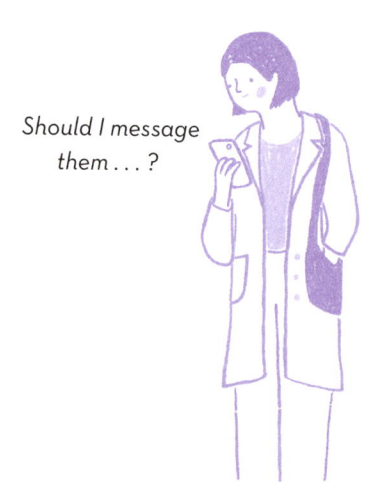

Should I message them...?

But when we do meet, our conversations skim the surface.

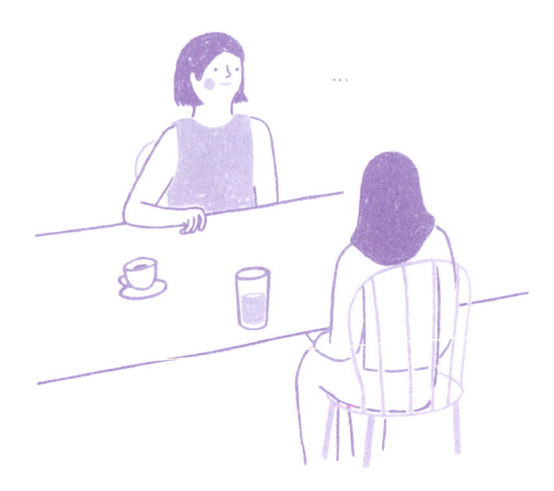

Only with a strange kind of distance.
A quiet emptiness.

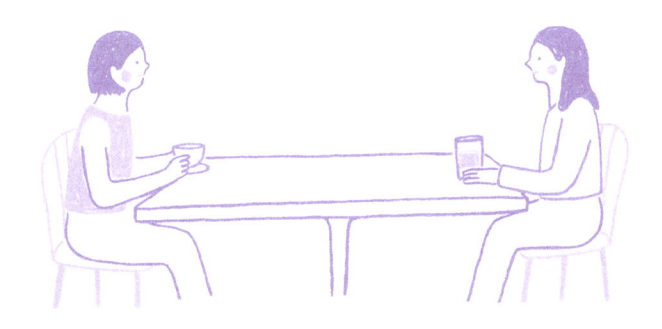

In that emptiness, only a faint sense of obligation
comes with the word 'friend'.

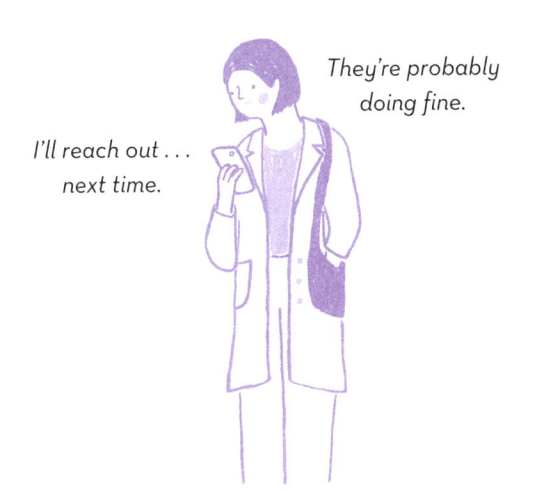

*I'll reach out . . .
next time.*

*They're probably
doing fine.*

I sometimes feel a quiet discomfort about not seeing my old friends as often. Is it guilt? Regret? Disappointment? It's hard to define this emotion. But of all the emotions I could be feeling, longing isn't one of them.

I'm not saying I don't miss them at all – but the feeling I do have is closer to nostalgia for a time we once shared, not for who we are to each other now.

The world praises those who hold on to long-standing relationships. Sometimes, that makes me wonder if I've failed at something important in life. We age, change and live differently, so it's natural that emotional distance grows, too. Still, this vague sense of obligation weighs heavily at times. I try to make time to see them now and then. But when we part ways, a hollow ache lingers – a quiet doubt. There are so many people I should see, but not many I want to.

After all, friendship isn't always about how long you've known someone. So I've decided not to cling too tightly to the years, the memories, the effort already spent. Whether it's an old friend or a new one, what matters most is how we feel now. Which relationships we choose to treasure – that's up to each of us.

As for me, I'd like to spend more time with people I can share joy with, fully and freely. After all, life is short. We only get one.

56
Meaning of Friendship

What is friendship?

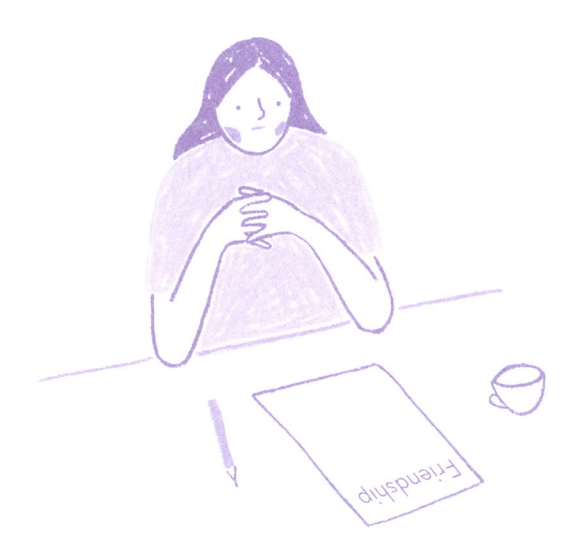

Even though we don't check in with them
every day, when we do,

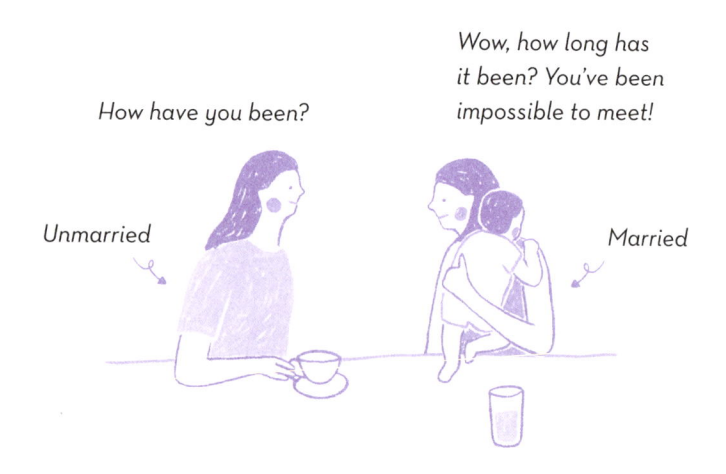

How have you been?

Wow, how long has it been? You've been impossible to meet!

Unmarried

Married

we give them our full attention with loud,
enthusiastic support.

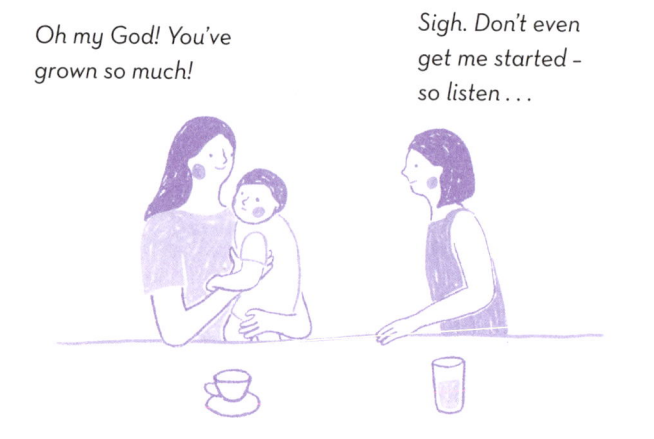

Oh my God! You've grown so much!

Sigh. Don't even get me started – so listen . . .

Seeing beauty in someone simply because your friend loves them.

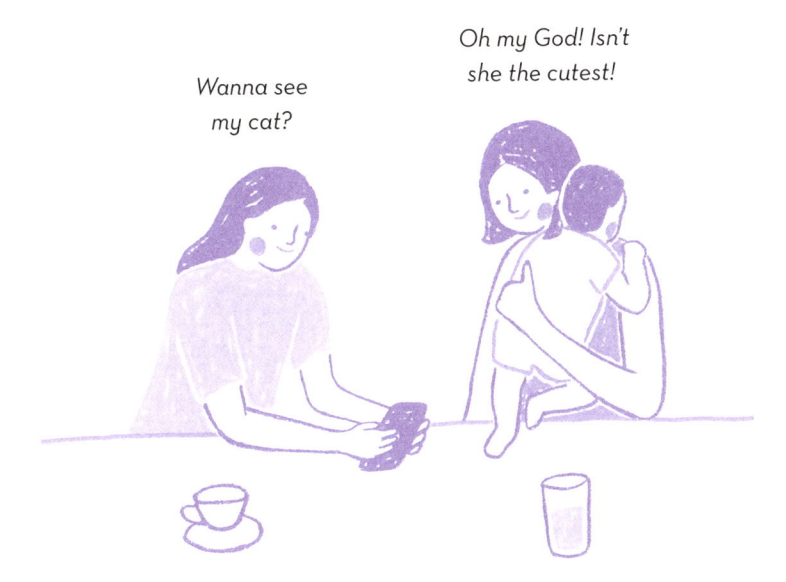

Wanna see my cat?

Oh my God! Isn't she the cutest!

57
People Always Need People

You always seemed capable and so independent,

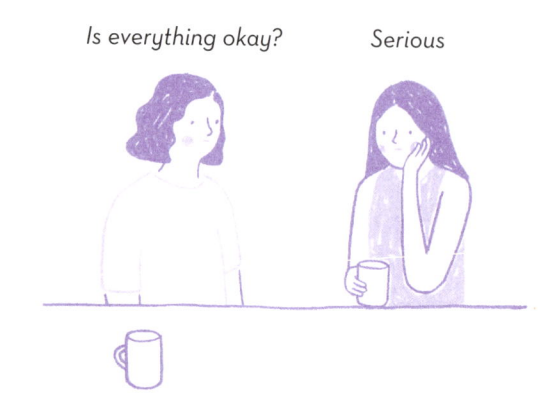

Is everything okay?

Serious

I thought you wouldn't even notice if I disappeared.

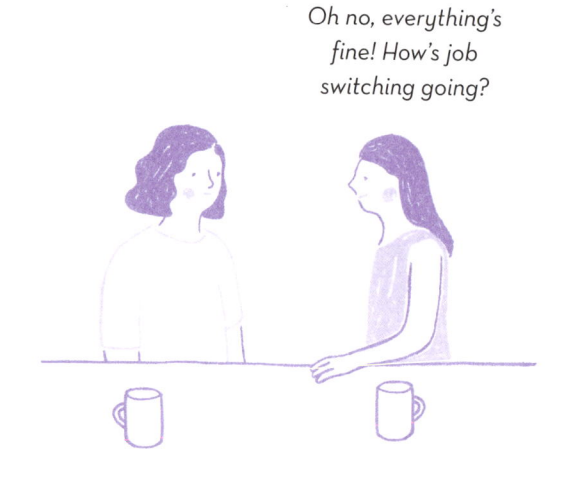

Oh no, everything's fine! How's job switching going?

But now I realise that you were just preparing yourself
for the hurt of being left alone.

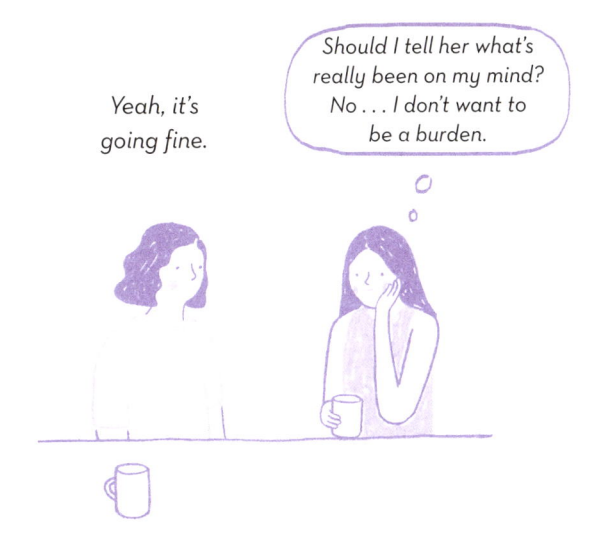

Yeah, it's going fine.

Should I tell her what's really been on my mind? No . . . I don't want to be a burden.

Turns out, you needed someone too –
and that someone was me.

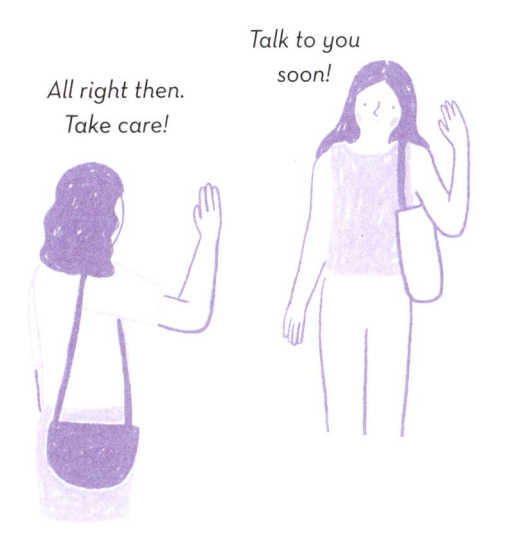

All right then. Take care!

Talk to you soon!

I had a friend who always seemed strongly independent. We'd known each other for a long time, but I never felt truly close to her. She never opened up about her struggles and rarely asked for help. She seemed to handle everything on her own, so I assumed she didn't really need me.

But over time – maybe it was age that had a way of softening us – things began to shift. We started sharing thoughts and feelings we never had before. And I realised, she *did* want to lean on someone. She had just been trying to grow stronger on her own in relationships she feared could end at any moment.

As we got closer, fear followed. Before, I didn't think I mattered, so nothing could really hurt. But now that I knew I mattered, I felt the weight of it. The feeling of having an effect on someone brings a quiet sense of responsibility.

Like people who care for something living – a plant, a pet – they may lose their sense of direction but rarely their sense of purpose. Because responsibility becomes a thread that connects us to life. Maybe that's why people often suggest that those struggling with depression try caring for something small, something alive.

Having an effect on another life – to matter to something beyond yourself – is a form of vitality. Without even realising it, we live by leaning on one another in ways both big and small.

Because in the end, we all need each other.

58
Taking a Step Back from Each Other's Lives

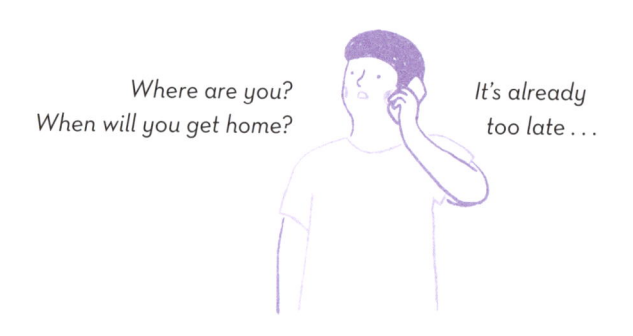

Where are you?
When will you get home?

It's already too late...

True love doesn't pry under the guise of care.

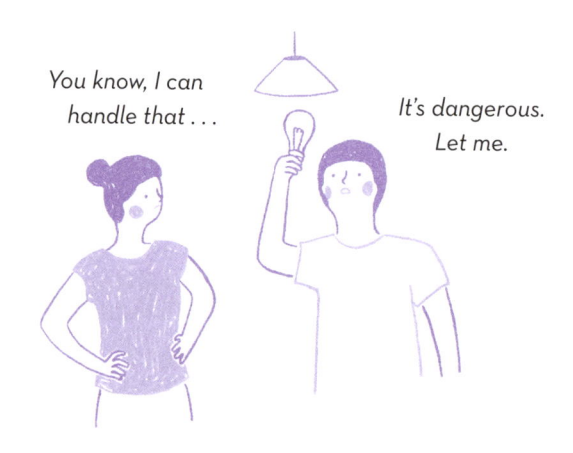

You know, I can handle that...

It's dangerous. Let me.

Or doing everything for them because you want to protect them.

*You're taking a class again?
I thought we'd spend the
weekend together...*

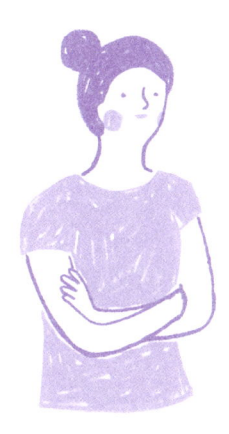

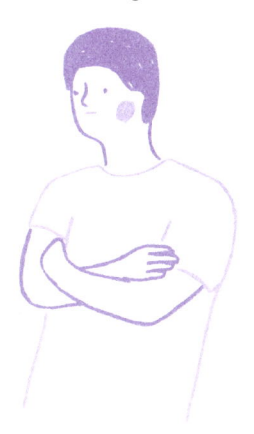

Maybe love, at its most sincere, is simply not making
the other person feel like they owe you.

Uncomfortable   *Guilty*

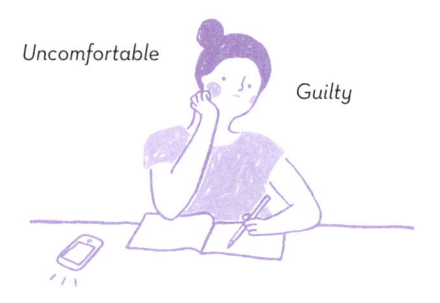

Maybe true love is about being able to do what you want for yourself

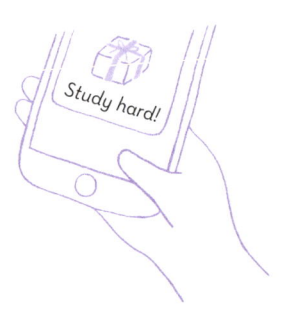

without either of you

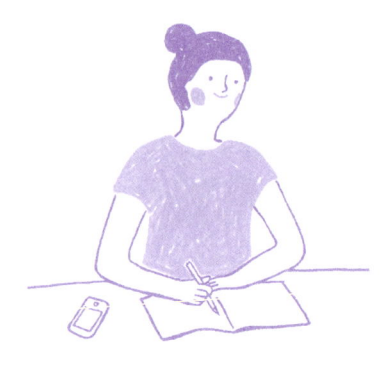

feeling sorry for it.

When we love someone, we tend to focus more on what we can give. We want to care, protect, cherish and support – to show love in all the ways we can. But in any relationship, we have to be careful of the quiet sense of entitlement that sometimes hides behind our giving. The desire to receive something in return for the love we give can lead us to believe we own a share in the other person's life. And when the other person senses this, they may begin to carry a lingering sense of debt, feeling that they must eventually repay all the love they've received.

Thoughts like, 'They've done so much for me', 'They've sacrificed so much' can cause us to prioritise the other person's feelings over our own decisions. We hesitate to make choices they might not agree with. We lose confidence in choosing what's right for our life. We tiptoe, unsure, weighed down by pressure we can't quite explain. Sometimes, we don't even try, because we assume they wouldn't approve.

When love becomes a way to quietly steer another person's life by planting seeds of guilt, that's no longer love. Instead of trying to give too much, maybe the healthier way is to step back, just a little, and focus on ourselves, too. From that space, love can breathe. And so can we.

MY LITTLE TIPS FOR BALANCING HEALTHY BOUNDARIES IN RELATIONSHIPS

For love to mean something, what we give must be grounded in mutual respect. Respect is not just an important part of healthy love – it's the foundation. The first step. And the one we must never forget.

59
The Timeless Kind of Magic

The things that never lose their magic with time
are often the simplest moments.

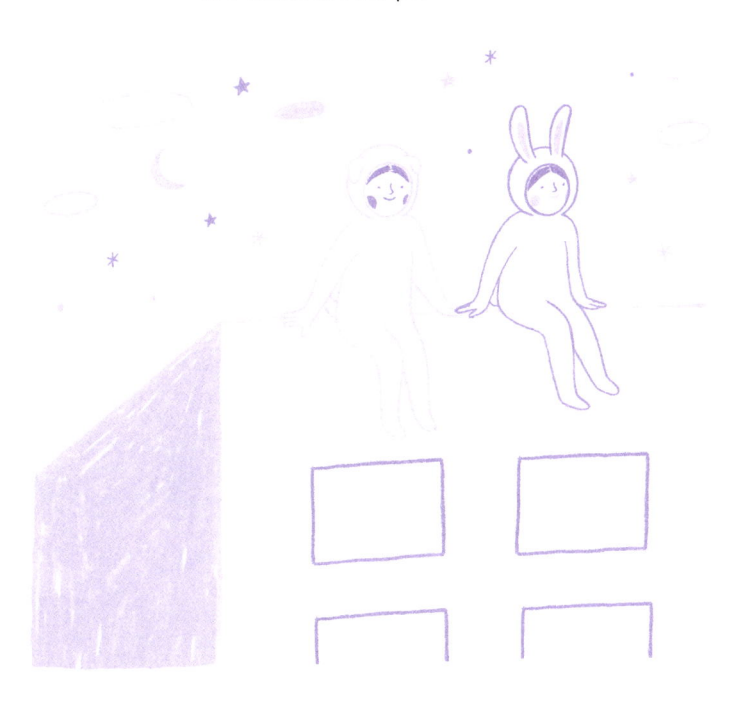

Your unique expression or little habit only I noticed.

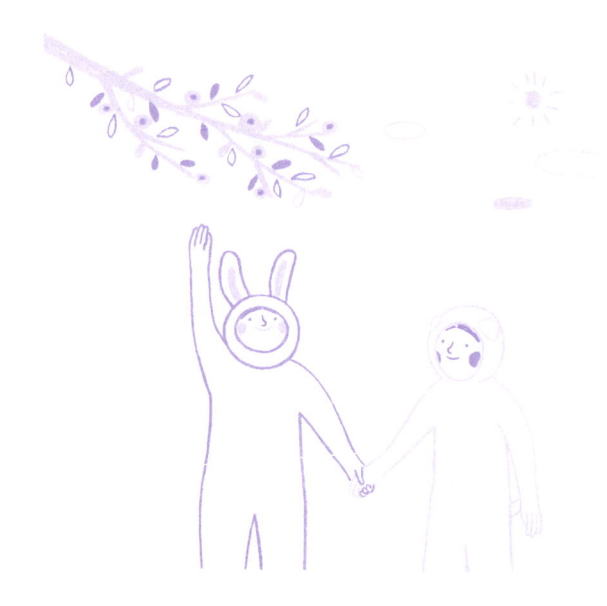

Our warm little moments.

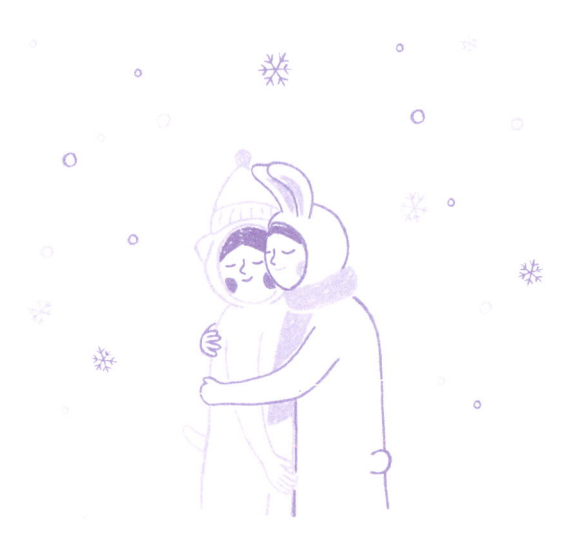

Even if those memories fade with time,

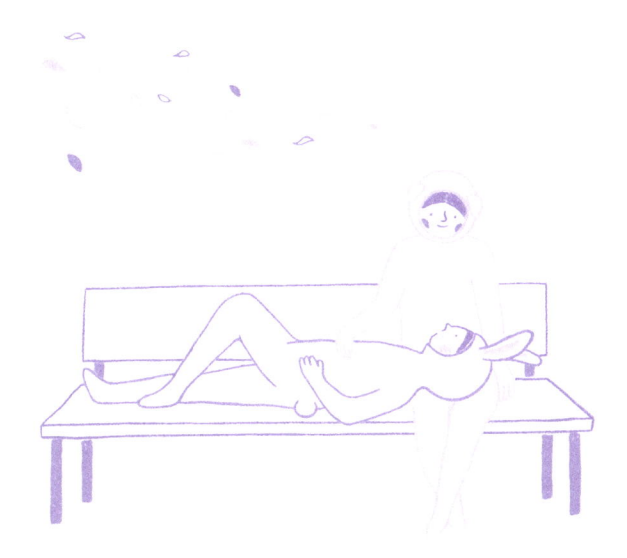

I know the way I felt back then was real
and will never fade.

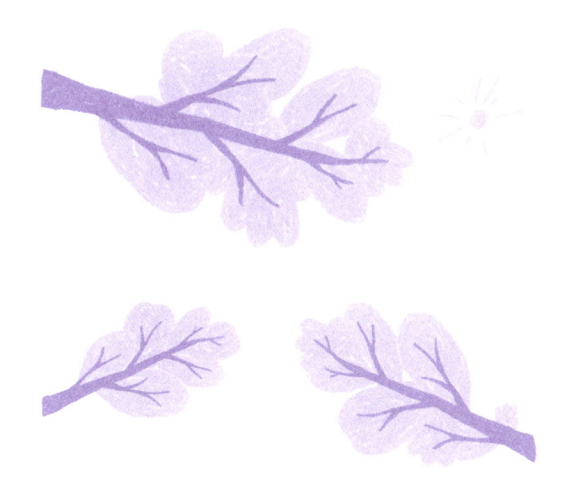

60
Relationship is Not a Means for Happiness

The presence of another person, on its own, can never be the ultimate key to happiness.

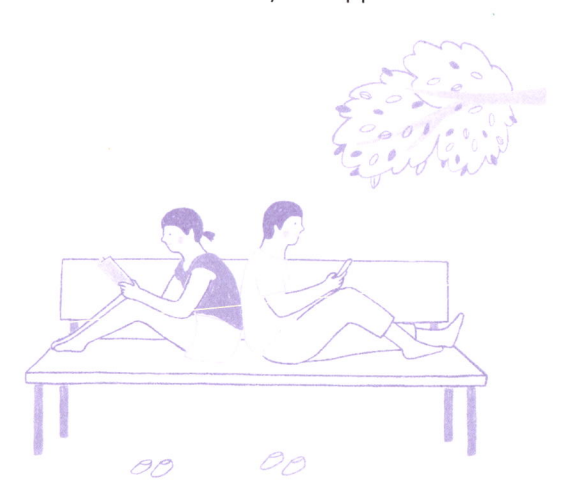

A supportive family, a loving partner, good friends – they can help, but they can't be everything.

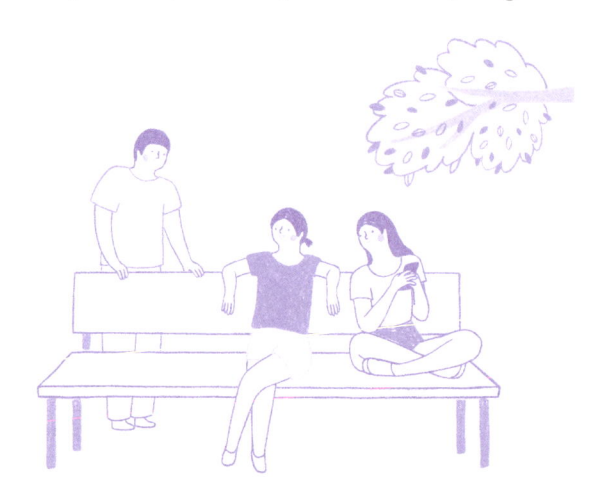

At the end of the day, we can only be as happy as we've decided we're willing to be.

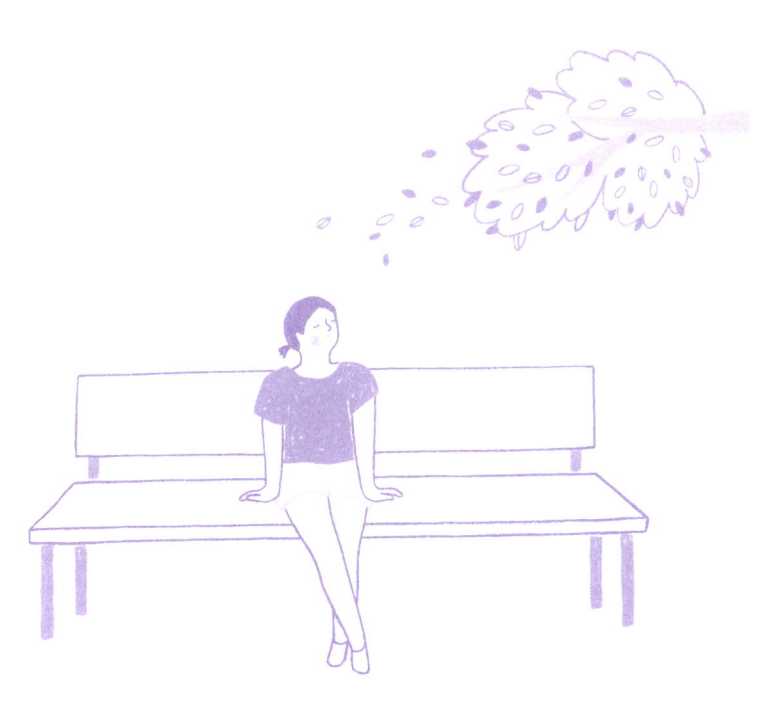

The human body is made up of about 70% water. So what makes up the other 30%? It feels like anxiety takes up that space for me. I've always been someone with a high 'anxiety index'. So relationships where I can openly share my worries without having to filter them are particularly special to me.

When I started drifting apart from a few close friends for various reasons, I thought my loneliness came simply from missing their presence. But looking back, I realised something surprising: even when we were together, I often felt alone. In a crowd, with a partner, even with family, the people closest to me – I still felt a certain kind of loneliness. If you've ever felt lonelier with people than you did on your own, you'll understand what I mean.

What I've come to realise is that the presence or absence of a person doesn't define my happiness. Looking more closely, the feeling I had wasn't loneliness from people leaving. It was the fear of losing the emotional safety that comes from sharing something deeply personal – for me, that was anxiety. For others, it might be something else.

Being with someone can definitely offer a sense of stability. While we can't expect another person to fill the deepest gaps within us, still, as social beings, there's a unique comfort that only connection and empathy can bring.

Ultimately, my happiness is my own responsibility. But within relationships, I can build it more fully. And maybe knowing that and truly accepting it is the key to coexisting more peacefully with the people I love.

61
How the Food Tasted, or the Breeze Smelled

I once remembered an incredibly delicious meal

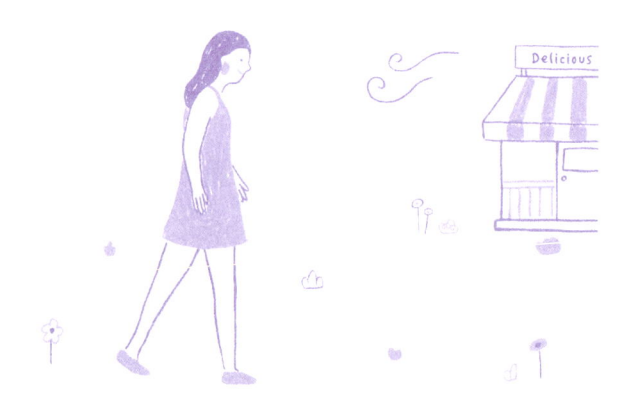

and only later realised what made it so special was the person I shared it with.

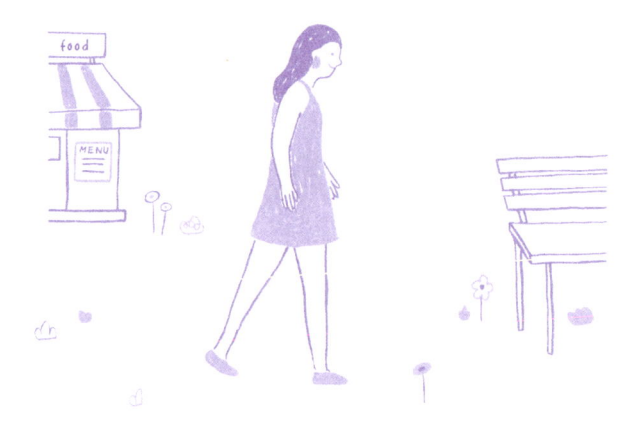

Our memories are deeply tied to our senses,

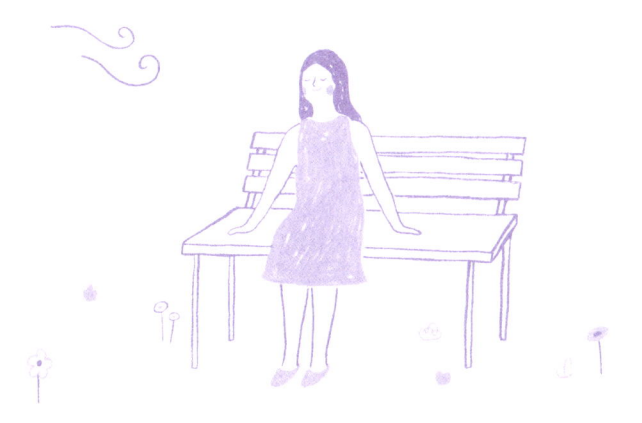

the taste of food or the scent of a breeze
doesn't just bring back moments, but the people
we shared them with.

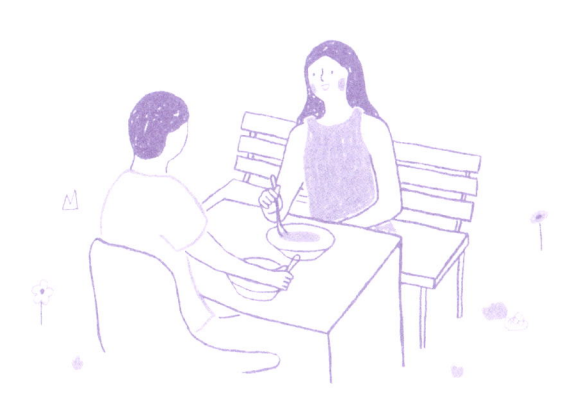

62
We're So Alike!

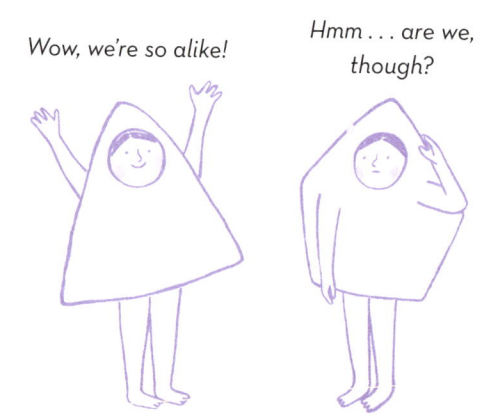

Wow, we're so alike! *Hmm... are we, though?*

We're all experts at finding similarities with people we like.

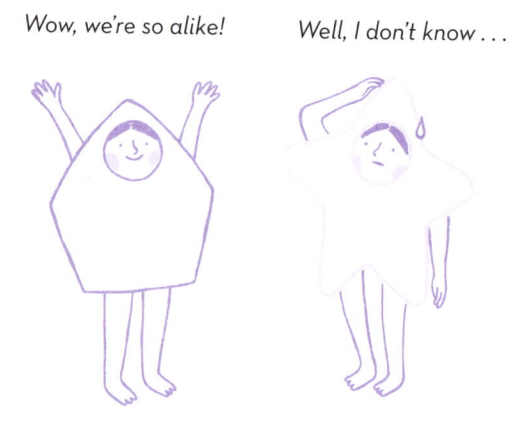

Wow, we're so alike! *Well, I don't know...*

Even if, in truth, we probably have more differences than things in common.

I think I'm more like Circle. We're soulmates.

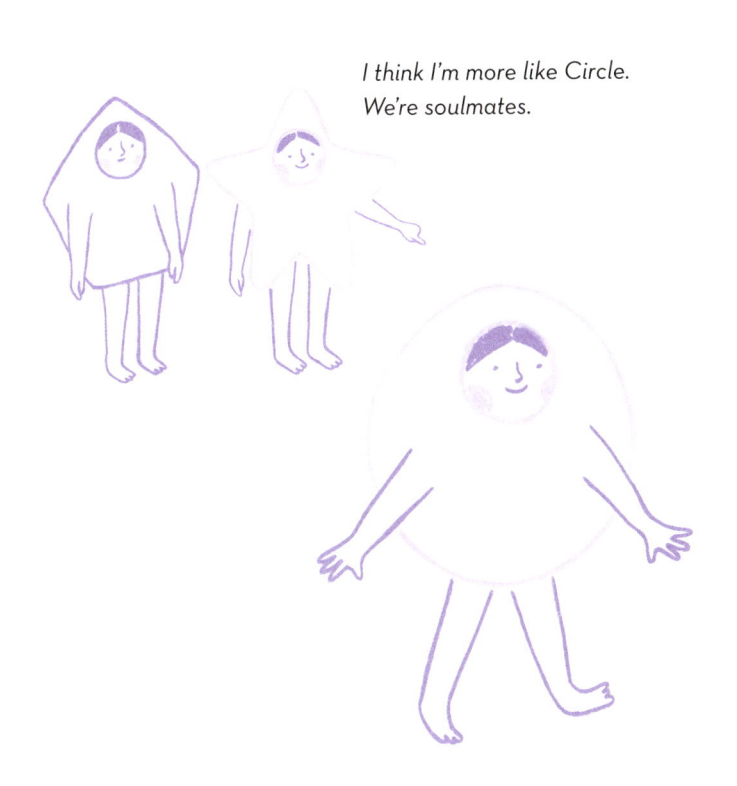

Maybe when we say, 'We're so alike!'

what we really mean is, 'I want to share more of myself with you.'

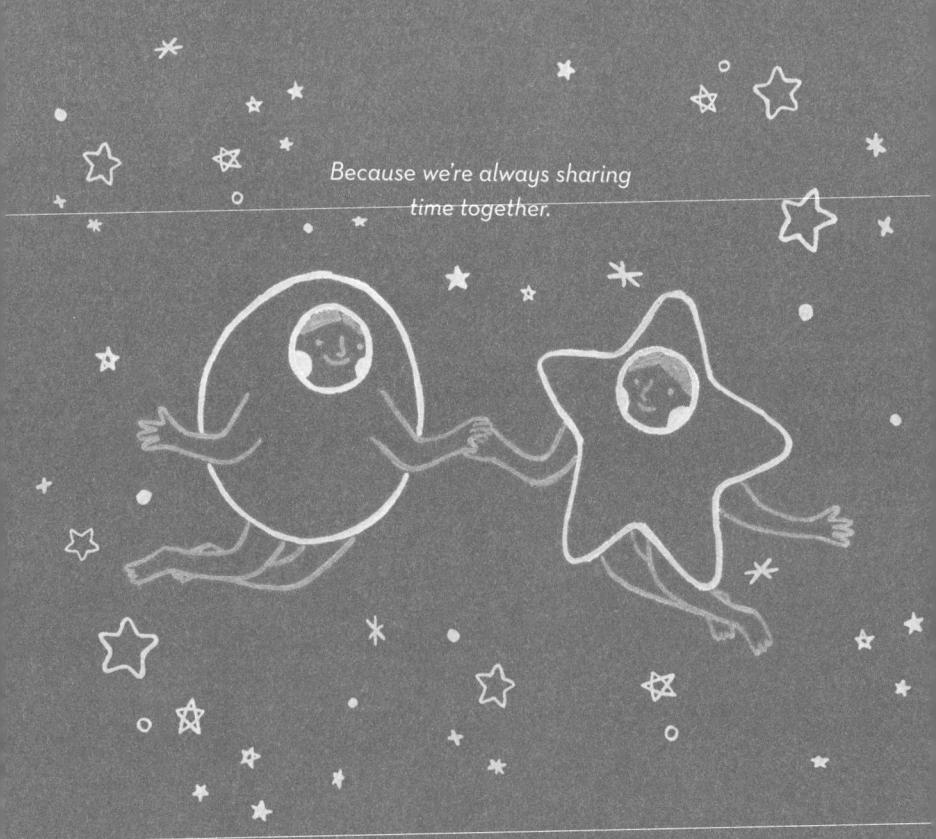

Because we're always sharing time together.

In the American movie 500 *Days of Summer*, the main character Tom develops a crush on his co-worker, Summer. When he finds out that she likes the same band as he does, he instantly believes they're destined to fall in love. That's when his younger sister says, 'Just because she likes the same bizarre crap you do doesn't mean she's your soulmate.'

We often attach meaning to small similarities with someone we like. Not because they're inherently significant, but because we want to share something with them. When we say, 'Our chemistry just clicks,' it's often nothing more than a quiet hope whispered inward: 'I like you. I want us to be close. I want even our differences to feel like a match.'

The idea of a soulmate, when you really think about it, is more abstract than we'd like to admit – a beautiful illusion we often project onto others because we want to believe in something magical. What's interesting is that when we like someone, we look for ways we're the same. When we dislike someone, we search for every possible difference. And even a few shared traits can be dismissed, just to confirm our discomfort.

It's funny how our perception of similarity or difference is often shaped not by facts, but by how we feel. So, when you find yourself noticing all the ways someone is 'different', it might just mean you feel uneasy around them, and that's okay.

A little distance might be what you need. And when someone seems remarkably similar to you, before you rush to call it fate, maybe start by simply acknowledging how much you like them. But don't spend too long wondering if they're the one. You might miss the moment.

63
There Are So Many Things More Important than Food

We all tend to project our own sense of lack onto others,

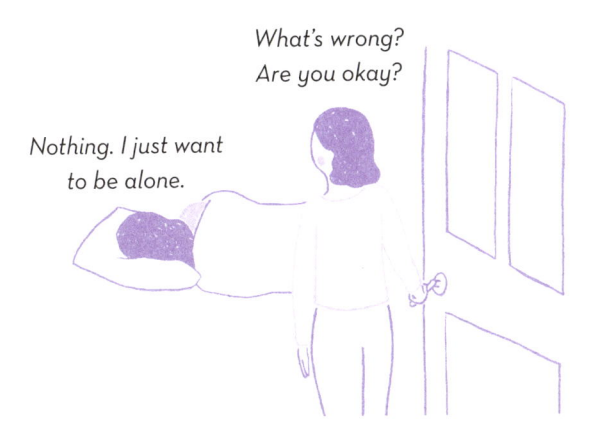

What's wrong? Are you okay?

Nothing. I just want to be alone.

and we assume they must need what we once needed.

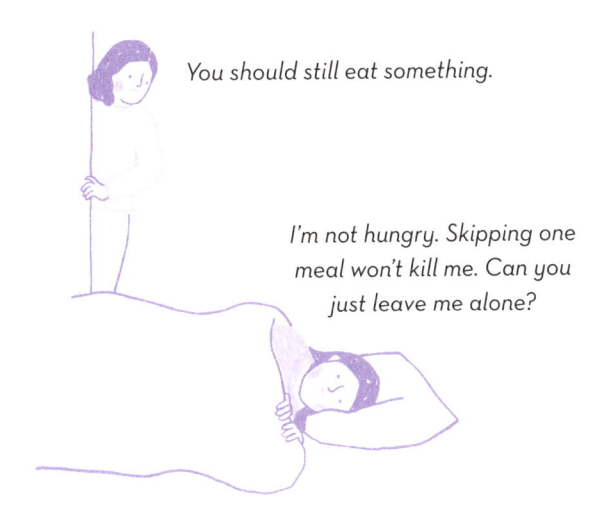

You should still eat something.

I'm not hungry. Skipping one meal won't kill me. Can you just leave me alone?

In doing so, we often miss what they truly need.

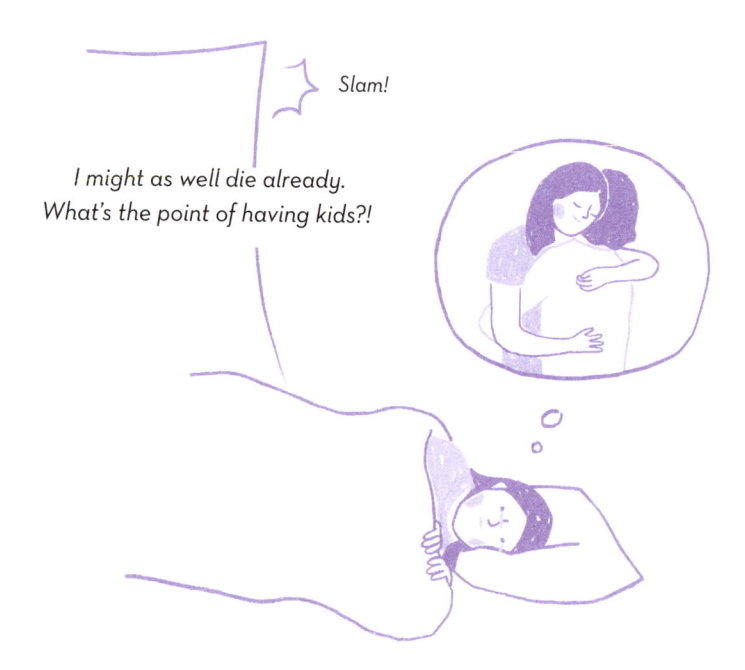

Slam!

I might as well die already. What's the point of having kids?!

But we know we truly care for each other.

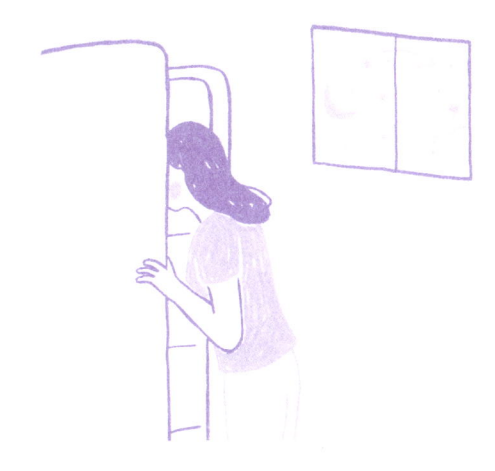

So why is it so hard to let each other know?

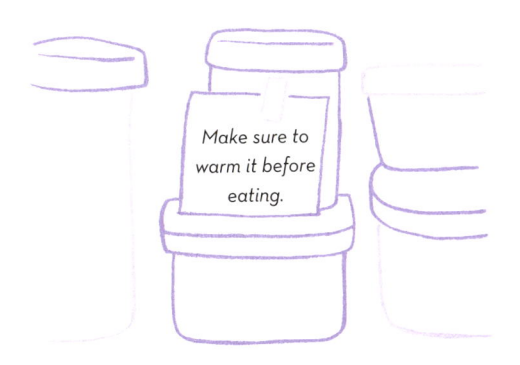

Make sure to warm it before eating.

In Korea, we often say to our friends, 'Have you been eating well?' or 'Let's grab a meal sometime' as a casual way of checking in. It's familiar, even comforting. But truthfully, I don't think I've ever really worried about whether they were eating well. It's probably only my parents who genuinely cared whether I'd eaten. They say people tend to give others what they themselves lacked while growing up. For a generation that knew hunger, a full meal meant care. So they pass that on to the people they love. But for me, there are many things in this world far more urgent than whether I've eaten today. Sometimes, more than a bowl of rice, I wish for a quiet word of understanding. More than a table full of dishes, a simple, silent hug.

Everyone carries a different kind of hunger. Some crave achievement. Others, recognition. Some hunger for love. And naturally, we look at others through the lens of what we've lacked. That's why, even with the best intentions, our comfort sometimes misses the mark. It's only human to interpret the world through our own experience, because it's the only lens we've ever known.

Still, every now and then, it might be worth opening our hearts to the world reflected in the gaze of someone we love.

In doing so, maybe we'll discover an entirely new way to love.

64
Letting Go of the Weight of Empty Connections

I no longer want to hold on to relationships that feel empty or obligatory.

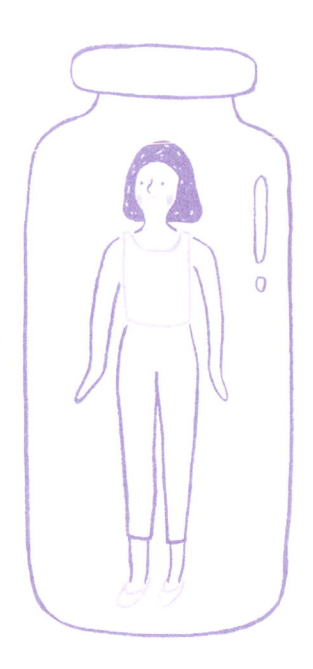

Ties kept out of habit – because 'you never know how things might turn out',

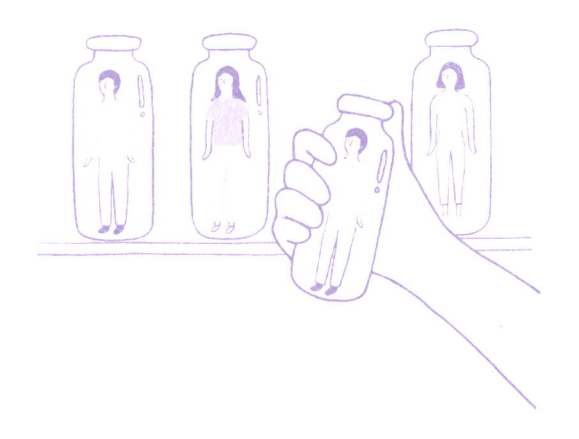

or 'I might need help one day' – are no longer worth the weight they carry.

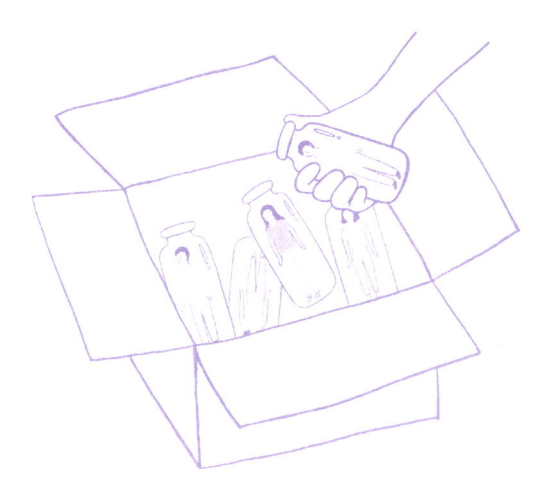

I've decided to let them go.

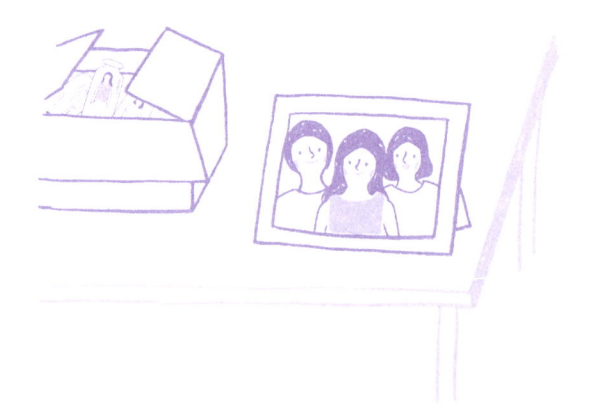

Because I've come to realise that what matters most
are the people who are truly here with me – now.

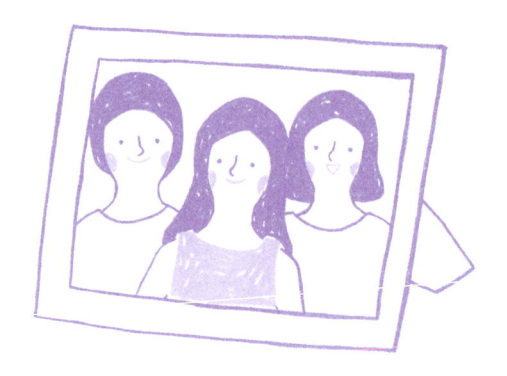

Some friendships fade without warning. Even people I used to be close with drifted away as we each focused on our own lives. Some stayed – the kind you catch up with now and then, sharing old stories, warm laughter. But others disappeared completely once jobs, marriages and kids took centre stage. Sometimes, it felt like I'd been erased from their world. And yes – it stung.

There was a time in my early adulthood, especially around the so-called 'marriage age', when I felt overwhelmed by the shallowness of relationships. I grew weary of people who reached out only during moments of celebration with messages that felt on the nose and meaningless. With their major life events like getting a job, switching careers, getting married and having a child, my relationships were quietly re-evaluated. One by one, I sifted through the people I used to know, gradually letting go of the weight of connections that no longer held meaning. They say the people who show up at just the right time – they're the ones who are meant to stay. Maybe friendships work that way, too.

In the end, there's only so much time, energy and emotional space one person can offer. So, all we can really do is accept that relationships shift with each season of life and pour our hearts into those who are still here, by our side.

MY LITTLE TIPS FOR BALANCING HEALTHY BOUNDARIES IN RELATIONSHIPS

Does the length of time you've known someone always reflect the depth of your relationship?
Not necessarily. What truly matters isn't how long they've been in your life, but how deeply they're felt – not in presence, but in connection.

65
Simple Words But Full of Heart

If there's one thing to understand before falling in love,

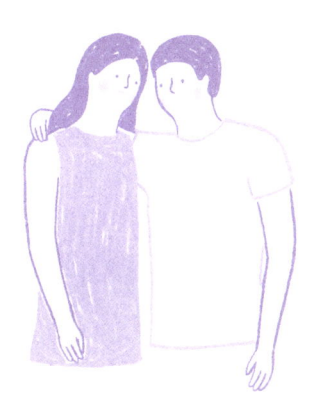

it is that people make promises they cannot keep when they speak of love.

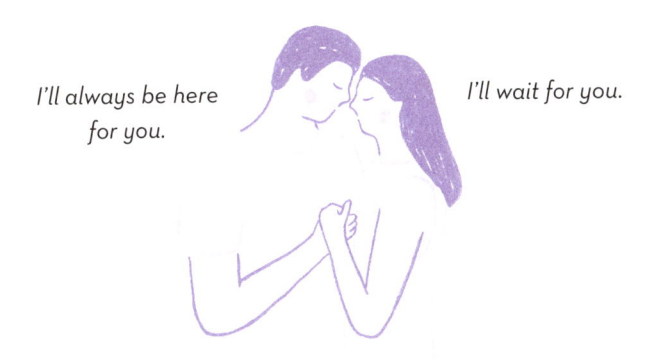

I'll always be here for you.

I'll wait for you.

But one thing worth remembering

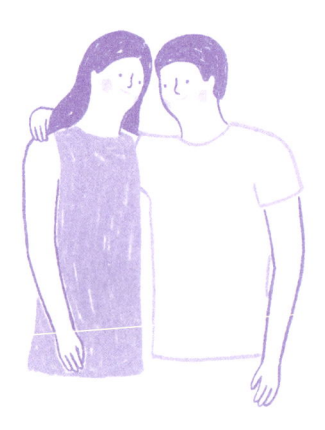

is that all those promises were, at the very least, sincere in that moment.

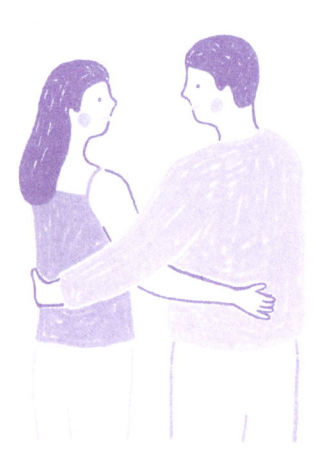

Because sometimes, when you can't show everything in your heart, you try your best to say it instead.

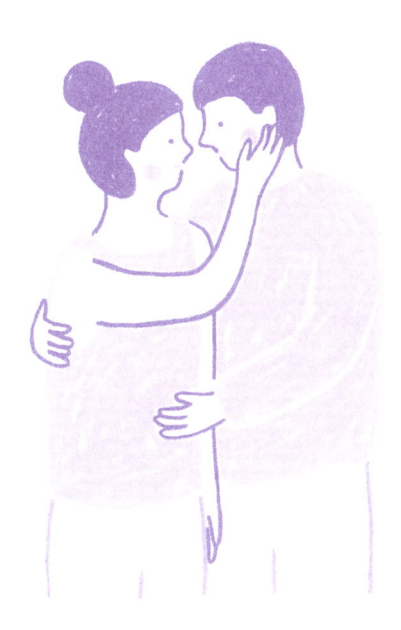

66
Expanding Our Universe

I had a misconception about intimacy for a long time, because of the misunderstanding of a scene from a film I saw during my school days – *Hedwig and the Angry Inch*.

There's a music video in the film, *Origin of Love*, which tells the story of how humans once had two heads, four arms and four legs, until the gods split them in half. And ever since, love has been about finding the other half, becoming whole again by sharing love and even pain.

And I took it the wrong way. For years, I believed that intimacy meant someone entering my fixed life – a one-sided process where I had to give up half of myself. It felt like losing space, losing shape, like everything would have to change. And that thought terrified me.

But we each live in our own universe – one that holds our preferences, values, quirks, personalities and routines. So, when two universes come into contact, there are bound to be collisions, big and small. It can be uncomfortable. Even painful.

But in that contact, something new happens. You experience what you never would have alone; you find intersections and shared meaning and you learn to hold space for difference. With every inch of connection, your emotional and mental landscape grows.

Recently, I learned about something called *crown shyness* - a phenomenon where trees of the same species grow close together, yet their branches never touch, leaving visible gaps between their canopies. No one knows exactly why these neighbouring trees keep a respectful distance, as if to avoid crowding or harming one another, growing side by side with care.

But watching them - respectfully close yet never invasive - I began to understand what it means to live in harmony, to grow together while still remaining whole.

To expand each other's worlds without consuming them.

67
Someone to Hold a Broken Piece of Your Heart

Who we truly need is not someone
perfect and whole,

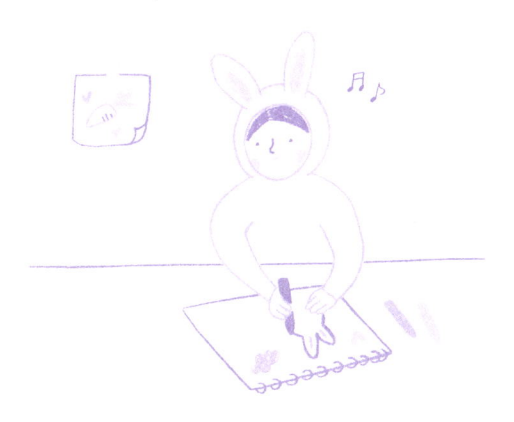

but someone who, even when you're broken,

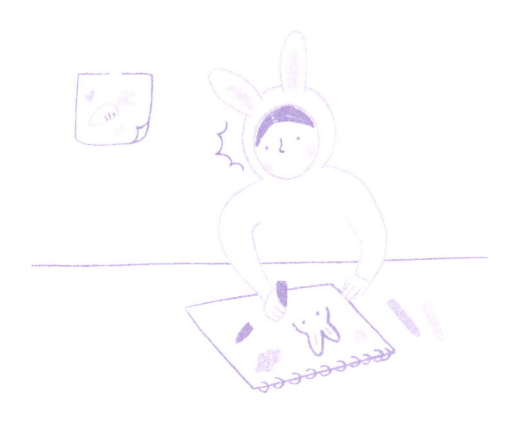

will still pick up a broken piece of your heart

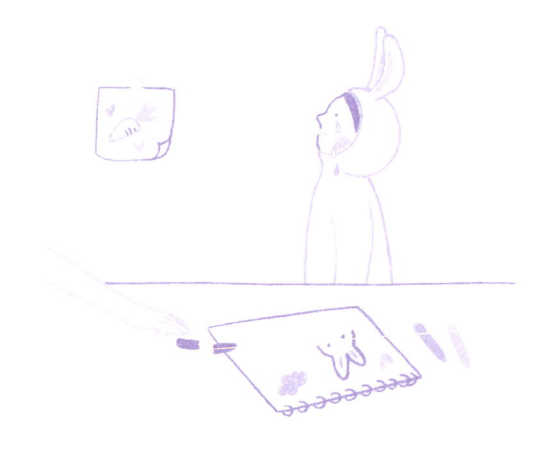

and stay with you through it all.

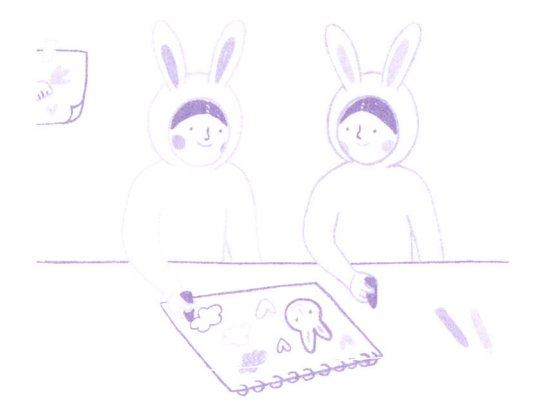

Before I became a full-time freelancer, I worked as an art instructor. There was one student who had to arrange the coloured pencils in the exact order of the rainbow. And if the colouring slipped outside the lines or her art tool broke, she'd burst into tears, completely overwhelmed. She reminded me of myself as a child. The anxiety. The need for control. Naturally, I grew attached to her and wanted to teach her well – not just art, but how to be gentle with oneself.

Over the years, she slowly began to change. When something upsetting happened, she'd come to me and say, 'It's okay.' One day, as she was colouring, a pastel stick snapped in two. She paused, then looked up at me and said: 'It's okay. Now I have two! We can colour together.'

Sometimes, comfort doesn't come from those who try to make us whole. Sometimes, what we need most is someone who can simply sit with us in our brokenness.

ABOUT THE AUTHOR

Dancing Snail is an acclaimed illustrator and writer. She is the illustrator of the bestselling Korean edition *I Want to Die but I Want to Eat Tteokbokki*. Having experienced depression, anxiety and burnout, she seeks to spread messages of compassion and patience to all those who feel burdened. She is based in South Korea.

ABOUT THE TRANSLATOR

Sandy Joosun Lee is a Korean-to-English translator based in Seoul. She studied Literature/Writing in University of California, San Diego. Her translations include Won-pyung Sohn's *Almond* and Miye Lee's *DallerGut Dream Department Store* duology. She also works in animation, translating and developing animated content, which includes *The Witcher: Nightmare of the Wolf* (2021) and *Star Wars: Visions* (2023).